Cultural Conceptions

Cultural Conceptions

On Reproductive Technologies and the Remaking of Life

Valerie Hartouni

 University of Minnesota Press

Minneapolis

London

Chapter 3 first appeared in a different form in *camera obscura* 29 (1992), copyright 1992 Indiana University Press, reprinted with the permission of Indiana University Press. Chapter 4 was originally published in *Provoking Agents: Gender and Agency in Theory and Practice*, ed. Judith Kegan Gardiner. Copyright 1995 by the Board of Trustees of the University of Illinois, used with permission from the University of Illinois Press. Chapter 5 first appeared in a different form in *Configurations* 1 (1994), used by permission of The Johns Hopkins University Press.

Published by the University of Minnesota Press
111 Third Avenue South, Suite 290, Minneapolis, MN 55401-2520
Printed in the United States of America on acid-free paper

Library of Congress Cataloging-in-Publication Data

Hartouni, Valerie.
    Cultural conceptions : on reproductive technologies and the
  remaking of life / Valerie Hartouni.
        p.   cm.
    Includes bibliographical references and index.
    ISBN 0-8166-2622-7 (hc : alk. paper). — ISBN 0-8166-2623-5
  (pbk. : alk. paper)
    1. Human reproductive technology—Social aspects.   2. Human
  reproductive technology—Moral and ethical aspects.   I. Title.
    [DNLM: 1. Reproduction Techniques.   2. Fetus—United States—
  legislation.   3. Abortion, Legal—United States.   4. Surrogate
  Mothers.   5. Culture.   6. Socioeconomic Factors.   WQ 208 H334c
  1997]
  RG133.5.H383   1997
  176—dc21
  DNLM/DLC
  for Library of Congress   96-39562

for *Lauren*

Surely there are in everyone's life certain connections, twists and turns which pass awhile under the category chance, but at the last, well examined, prove to be the very Hand of God.

SIR THOMAS BROWNE, *Religio Medici*

Contents

Acknowledgments

Many people have had a hand in making this book possible in all its various forms and moments. Although I completed a dissertation on the contemporary abortion debate in the mid-1980s, my attention to reproductive discourses in a somewhat fuller sense began sometime later with a phone call from Constance Penley asking me to contribute an essay on the new reproductive technologies to a collection she and Andrew Ross were editing. That essay—which appears in this book as chapter 2—marked the beginning of my fascination with the workings of contemporary reproductive discourses and constitutes the basis for the inquiries that together constitute this study. To Constance, then, I feel a special debt of gratitude. I feel an equally deep sense of gratitude toward Wendy Brown, who, if the truth be told, had to persuade me to return Constance's call in the first place, so convinced was I that she had called the wrong number. Many drafts and lifetimes have since filled the years and throughout both Wendy has been a spirited interlocutor and mostly fearless friend.

Other friends and colleagues have offered conversation and life-sustaining camaraderie along the way as well as many good suggestions for revising chapters of this book, even if I have been a somewhat recalcitrant recipient of their good advice. This community of extraordinary people includes my colleagues at UC San Diego, in particular, Vince Raphael, Michael Meranze, and Roddey Reid; Chris Littleton, who has tried to teach me something about how law works; and the late David Schneider, whose wry humor, sharp sense of irony, and intellectual agility contributed to typically interesting, often challenging, and occasionally warped exchanges. Similarly gifted people whose wit, sanity, insight, and compassion have shaped my world and work and lent both a lusciously rich texture include Sherri Paris, Thelma Francis, Gail Hershatter, Susan Kent, Katie King, Arnie Fischman, Adele Clarke, Sharon Traweek, Sarah Banet-Weiser, Susan Harding, Rusten Hogness, Tim Cook, Jack Yeager, and Dan Scripture. Donna Haraway has been a much-cherished teacher, colleague, and friend— someone who has gone the long way with only an occasional squawk and who has been in most every way and from the beginning, the difference in my life that has had a deep, profound, and lasting effect. Finally, what I have learned and continue to learn from Donna's work and changing vision as well as the politically incisive writings of Rosalind Petchesky, Rayna Rapp, Emily Martin, and Paula Treichler is truly immeasurable. I feel a deep appreciation for the keen intellect and generosity of each of these scholars and an especially deep respect for their unwavering commitment through the years to building and protecting sites of feminist research.

Paula Treichler, Lisa Cartwright, and Jane Bennett read the original version of the manuscript for the University of Minnesota Press, and each offered many valuable suggestions for sharpening the arguments, while Lisa Freeman and Carrie Mullen were editors of the first order: patient, enthusiastic, and thoroughly gracious at each stage of the long process of production. Alison Schapker did some of the trench work entailed in preparing the final version of the manuscript for publication, and I owe much to her fine eye for detail. Financial and institutional support for writing portions of this book were provided by the Susan B. Anthony Center at the University of Rochester, the Humanities Research Institute at the University of California, Irvine, and Academic Senate Research Grants from the University of California, San Diego.

Introduction

In 1993, the Supreme Court handed down a ruling in *Bray v. Alexandria Women's Health Clinic* the logic of which, although predictable in many respects, might nevertheless give even the most seasoned skeptic reason to pause and consider—indeed, marvel in disbelief at—how dramatically refigured the landscape that is abortion has become over the course of the past two decades. In this case, the Court was asked to determine whether the "rescue" demonstrations engaged in by anti-abortion activists at abortion clinics for the purpose of disrupting clinic operations deliberately deprive women seeking abortion (and related medical and counseling services) of their constitutionally protected right to interstate travel by making the destination of that travel inaccessible.[1] Although the Court ruled that such demonstrations *did not* infringe upon women's constitutional rights, what is striking about this case is not its outcome. What is striking is the reasoning that produced the Court's ruling, the notion, in other words, that anti-abortion demonstrations do not deprive women of having or exercising any constitutionally secured right or privilege because such demonstrations are conducted for the sole purpose of protecting abortion's "innocent victims," and thus *have nothing to do with women.*

Centrally at issue in *Bray* was the meaning and scope of the Civil Rights Act of 1871, and in particular, the first clause of the Reconstruction-era statute. Through a series of decisions handed down by

1

the Court in the intervening century or so, this clause had come to be interpreted as prohibiting activities among two or more persons (conspiracies) motivated by "some racial or perhaps otherwise class-based invidious discriminatory animus" and intended, either directly or indirectly, to deprive others of having and exercising their constitutionally protected rights and privileges. The question was whether this clause could be said to provide a federal cause of action against demonstrators who obstruct clinic access and operations. Or, re-posing and sharpening the question to bring more clearly into focus its stakes as the Court assessed them in *Bray*, Does opposition to abortion constitute a basic discriminatory attitude toward women in general? Are antiabortion demonstrations motivated by a discriminatory animus directed specifically at women and conducted for the purpose of impeding their protected right to interstate travel, affecting their conduct, or forcibly preventing them from exercising a right still guaranteed by *Roe v. Wade*?

Writing for the majority, Supreme Court Justice Antonin Scalia dismissed as absurd the notion that opposition to abortion—blockading clinic entrances, damaging clinic property, threatening and intimidating clinic clientele, and overwhelming local law enforcement—could "possibly be considered an irrational surrogate for opposition to (or paternalism towards) women."[2] As Scalia figured the matter, "the characteristic that formed the basis of the targeting . . . , was not womanhood, but the seeking of abortion."[3] Motivated by the desire to stop abortion and reverse its legalization, rescue operations, he argued, were simply that: "physical interventions between abortionists and the innocent victims of abortion" with the clear and ultimate goal of "rescuing" innocent human lives.[4] As such, they were not aimed at or defined with reference to women, nor could they be said to reflect a derogatory view of, an overtly hostile attitude toward, or a conscious, discriminatory intent with respect to them. "Whatever one thinks of abortion," Scalia argued, "there are common and respectable reasons for opposing it other than hatred of or condescension toward (*or indeed any view at all* concerning) women as a class."[5]

Any view at all? While recognizing that opposition to abortion is not, as Justice Stevens put it in his dissenting opinion, "ipso facto to discriminate invidiously against women," we might nevertheless be inclined, as was Stevens, to reconsider the obvious: only women have the capacity to become pregnant and thus to need or have an abortion.[6] In

this respect, abortion is and always has been a "uniquely female practice," a practice in which only women engage.[7] It is, moreover, a right
that only women possess and have the capacity to exercise, and one
might argue that it is precisely this capacity that is constrained or
thwarted when violence is used to intimidate women entering clinics.[8]
Finally—and this Stevens noted only furtively in his dissent—abortion
is an issue that has shaped and been shaped by a dense constellation of
questions and an equally dense set of cultural contests, in both this
century as well as the last, despite its shifting meanings having to do
with the control and containment of women's fertility and sexuality,
the terms and conditions of childbearing and child rearing, the meaning of motherhood and manhood, and the structure, meaning, and organization of the family as well as of gender, marriage, reproduction,
and heterosexuality.[9] If Operation Rescue claims—as it did in a 1990
editorial—that it is the rightful heir of the women's movement and
that its members have become "the true defenders of women in this
generation . . . [by] allowing women to be what God intended them to
be,"[10] how is it possible that they could, as Scalia maintains they do,
oppose abortion and not have "any view at all concerning women"?
What is the view that Scalia contends, and the majority of the Supreme
Court apparently agrees, is no view at all?

In each of the chapters in this book I proffer a response to this question and a range of others like it by interrogating the cultural crafting
and apparatuses of vision in the context of contemporary debates over
new and, in the case of abortion and some forms of surrogacy, not-so-
new reproductive practices and processes. Chapter 1 takes up the issue
of vision directly and begins by considering Olive Sacks's account of a
fifty-year-old man whose sight was restored through surgery after
forty-five years of blindness and who nevertheless was unable to
"see"—to make sense of the images and objects that appeared within
his field of vision. Using Sacks's account to develop the notion that
what we typically regard as contaminating vision is precisely its pre-
condition, I argue, following other cultural theorists, that "seeing" is a
thoroughly situated and mediated activity. Indeed, as Sacks's tale
forcefully illustrates, "The innocent eye is blind."[11] Seeing is a set of
learned practices, a set of densely structured and structuring interpretive practices, that engages us in (re)producing the world we seem to
apprehend only passively and, through such engagement, facilitates
the automatic, if incomplete, operation of power. Subsequent chapters

work from and complexify this initial discussion of vision or seek to discern more finely the multiple and often contradictory logics and operations of seeing—the theoretical underpinnings, grounding assumptions, and cultural stakes—that render both plausible and possible the many stories that now circulate in this late-twentieth-century North American moment about reproductive relations and relationships. Each chapter is occasioned by one of the many public controversies that erupted during the 1980s and early 1990s over the use of a new reproductive technology or one of several highly publicized disputes that ensued when alternative reproductive arrangements produced an excess of relationships that proved difficult to configure socially or to consolidate legally. The readings that follow in each, taken together, foreground, map, and critically scrutinize how legal, medical, scientific, and popular discourses work and have worked—more or less successfully—to manage the destabilizing effects and contain the destabilizing potential of alternative reproductive arrangements and relations, or keep intact a world that otherwise appears and is presumed to be self-evidently given.

In chapter 2, I sketch in broad strokes some of the constitutive components of the production of a new form and practice of life, the fetus-as-person, along with the subtle, sometimes not so subtle, and, in either case, significant shifts in the juridical position of women that both abetted and accompanied this production. The chapter opens with the Senate Judiciary Subcommittee hearings on the personhood status of the fetus. Conducted in 1981, these hearings were dismissed at the time by critics as a thoroughly transparent political ploy in which moral and theological arguments with respect to the question of fetal personhood were refigured as "science," or new discoveries in human embryology and the still nascent field of fetology. And, notwithstanding pretense, a clearly reactionary agenda was at play in eclipsing, at least partially, the vast chasm between what senators and scientists throughout the hearings seemed nevertheless to treat as comparable, interchangeable categories. However, through a frame that now spans nearly fifteen years, the effects of these hearings seem to me decidedly far-reaching. Although a dubious political ploy, clearly, they were as well a rhetorically masterful—because publicly persuasive—performance that proffered scaffolding for the subsequent, decade-long, reconstruction of who (or what) is a subject with legal standing. They represent a moment of great theater that would undoubtedly have passed into obscurity, but was instead repeatedly restaged throughout the culture and decade, bolstered by the momentum of a national backlash, animated by a cultural rescripting of the representational texts of difference, and augmented by the development and mainstream marketing of new reproductive innovations and interventions.

If the debate about abortion more or less initiates the discussion in chapter 2, abortion is nevertheless treated throughout the discussion as merely one reproductive technology that has shaped and has been shaped by the development and application of others. Extending the lens in this way or placing abortion in a larger discursive context provides a more richly textured rendering of the reproductive landscape of the 1980s. It works to highlight the powerful, constitutive influence of abortion discourse on how such issues as postmortem ventilation, fetal therapy and repair, infertility, in vitro fertilization, surrogacy, and ultrasound imaging—issues otherwise treated, publicly, as discrete— were substantively construed across the distinct but related arenas of law, medicine, science, and popular culture. It also throws into clear relief the resculpting effect that these new and, in some cases, experimental reproductive practices have had with respect to the meaning and public construction of abortion. When Supreme Court Justice Sandra Day O'Connor argued in a dissenting opinion in *Akron* that the trimester framework set out by Justice Blackmun in *Roe v. Wade* was "clearly on a collision course with itself" and "completely unworkable" because "fetal viability in the first semester of pregnancy may be possible in the not too distant future," the effect in this case of arresting visual images and widely publicized, highly sensationalized (and only rarely successful) obstetric techniques, is obvious.[12]

In chapter 3, I bring the contemporary debate about abortion more centrally and exclusively into focus or stage an examination of the shifting registers of cultural meaning that construct abortion through a close reading of a rhetorically rich nine-minute, ostensibly "prochoice" video, *S'Aline's Solution*. This 1991 video depicts one woman's struggle to come to terms with an aborted pregnancy and is particularly instructive in its use of what I argue is a distinctly post-1980s vernacular with respect to abortion. Reminiscent of videos produced by proponents and opponents of abortion throughout the 1980s, *S'Aline's Solution* adopts an aura of medical authority, largely through its use of bioscape imagery from Lennart Nilsson's widely acclaimed *Nova* documentary, *The Miracle of Life*. It ostensibly situates viewers "inside" the reproductive body as witnesses to what is clearly intended to be read as a saline abortion. And, finally, it participates in the moral rehabilitation of "choice" through a sobering performance of regret and the use of images of fetuses in utero—images drawn from Nilsson's *Miracle of Life* and identified by the video's voice-over as the child who "will never be child"—that together work to counter the antiabortion charge that women have abortions without thought and for trivial reasons. As in contemporary discourse and debate, even among those who champion "choice," *S'Aline's Solution* constructs abortion as a violent and traumatic interruption of natural processes or a grim and grievous choice. Although questions of sexual freedom and reproductive autonomy may haunt what the video artist insists is a "prochoice" text, these questions are eclipsed in the end by the more riveting story the video appears to present of innocence imperiled and innocence betrayed.

S'Aline's Solution occupies what are, in effect, prolife representations, meanings, and practices as the given of abortion and, in this occupation, both suggests and reveals, among other things, the degree to which prolife discourse has so saturated public debate as to now set its terms and seem part of the fabric of fact. The interesting question with respect to the video and other sites of cultural contest as well is whether images like the ones that have circulated in the context of the abortion dispute can be appropriated and oppositionally inflected. Can such images be shackled to narrate a story altogether different from the one they typically service and eventually seem self-evidently to tell? I argue that, at least in the case of the video, the strategy of re-inflection fails, so great is the undertow of signification that surrounds the bioscape imagery and, in particular, the image of the free-floating fetal form. And what underwrites and forcefully sustains this claim is the curious—some might say perverse—"fact" that the sequence of images in the video that audiences consistently read as depicting a saline abortion are "actually" images, again drawn from Nilsson's *Miracle of Life*, of ejaculation. Although viewers embark on an excursion of discovery at the opening of *S'Aline's Solution*, it is an altogether different kind of excursion than they have been led to believe they are on. Indeed, what viewers encounter is not a life-and-death drama as it naturally unfolds, but a (social) text and one whose story they are not just passively reading, but actively constructing.

In chapters 4 and 5, I shift the focus of analysis to consider the practice of surrogacy, or "contract pregnancy" as it is sometimes called, to foreground the otherwise elided presence of the market in relations that have traditionally been regarded as "outside" wage labor and commercial production.[13] Scholars disciplinarily situated in sociology, law, women's studies, political science, and anthropology have written in clear, precise, and often persuasive ways about surrogacy's commercial underpinnings, its potential for exploitation, and its similarities to prostitution, as well as its value in expanding reproductive choice and thus freedom. On other fronts, considerable attention has been devoted to developing policy with respect to the practice and to determining whether and in precisely what ways it should be regulated.[14] In the interest of avoiding confusion, I should say at the outset that what I find compelling about the controversy that surrounds this alternative reproductive arrangement has little to do with questions of commercialization and policy formation or with the legislative breast-beating that periodically transpires in the acrimonious, anxiety-ridden moment of a breached contract. What I find particularly interesting and worth pausing over—indeed, what is scrutinized in chapters 4 and 5— is the way in which the courts have attempted both to make sense of and to metabolize the practice.

In chapter 4 I proffer a critical examination of the infamous 1987 New Jersey case of Baby M, and in chapter 5 I examine the somewhat less well-known, but no less striking, 1991 California case of Anna Johnson. In both chapters I take a considered look at the constellation of narratives the courts deployed in these cases and the multiple translations in which they engaged not merely to referee but, in some more fundamental sense, to make legible surrogacy's deeply unsettling if also inescapable "excesses" within existing understandings and structures of kinship.[15] Judge Sorkow in the Baby M case and Judge Parslow in the case of Anna J were both faced with the clearly formidable task of explaining how it was that the pregnant body was not also—or at least need not be considered as—the real maternal body. Indeed, both judges were called upon to decipher how it was that the pregnant body could be an instrument of monogamous heterosexual union and thus nature and, at the same time, a decidedly unnatural, utterly extraneous, and potentially menacing constituent of that union once it had performed its function.

How was this body to be made sense of and accounted for, and by what name would it be called? Or, situating these questions within the frame of the court, what cultural texts scripted and were transmitted through Sorkow's finding that Mary Beth Whitehead—a high school dropout and former sex worker—was merely a "viable vehicle" for the fulfillment of Bill Stern's constitutionally protected right to procreate and "unfit," in any event, to raise a child to whom she was related genetically, but to whom, in his reading, she bore no "maternal" tie? And, asking now a similar question of Judge Parslow's ruling, What cultural narratives underwrote and *made plausible* the judge's claim that Johnson's only tie to the white baby she had gestated, but with whom she shared no genetic link, was, at best, that of a "foster parent," analogous to, but no more significant, socially, than the kind of provisional bond he imagined a wet nurse might form with her charge?[16] Finally, with respect to both cases, what social worlds and relations rendered surrogacy legally and culturally legible and, in rendering it legible, were themselves reproduced?

That each of the rulings worked, in the end, to safeguard the prerogatives of race and class privilege seems to me, in some sense, both obvious and given—preserving these prerogatives is part of the containment project entailed in both interrupting and regulating the proliferation of meanings, identities, and relationships generated by the panoply of new reproductive practices. The interesting and important challenge, I would argue, lies in tracking how such entitlements and the systems of classification that organize them are produced as matters of natural fact—indeed, how in the context of the surrogacy rulings the pregnant body is *produced* as self-evidently parasitical and *in that production* becomes yet again and yet another (kind of) instrument of reproduction.

Chapter 6 constitutes what I think of as the transitional moment in this book. With the questions raised at the end of chapter 5 concerning Anna Johnson's custody bid and "black maternal nature" framing its discussion, chapter 6 functions as well as a kind of preamble to the analysis I develop in the final chapter organized around what Sarah Franklin has characterized as the culture's current romance with genes.[17] Chapter 6 moves on from surrogacy to consider the set of responses that swiftly followed the 1994 publication of *The Bell Curve*, an eight-hundred-page tome by the late Richard Herrnstein and Charles Murray in which the authors link social stratification to genetically rooted differences in cognitive capacity. More specifically and, for that matter, accurately, in this chapter I pause over the disturbing lack of response amid volumes of otherwise exercised commentary to what occupies the good middle third of the book—to wit, Herrnstein and Murray's arguments regarding black women's fertility and out-of-wedlock births as well as the authors' eugenically motivated recommendations for both regulating and rehabilitating the reproductive black female body.

I argue that, notwithstanding the more obvious and obviously incendiary issue of IQ, the primary object of Herrnstein and Murray's ire, and the primary subject of their book, is what they regard as the federally subsidized procreative excesses of self-evidently promiscuous black women. Black women's bodies emerge in their text as the site and source of social pollution, cultural degeneracy, mental deficiency, and genetic incapacity, and it is on, in, and through these bodies that they insist social policy must be performed. As Murray put the matter in a 1993 editorial for the *Wall Street Journal*, "Single women with children are a drain on the community's resources and in larger numbers destroy a community's capacity to sustain itself."[18] Although commentators have taken critical aim at *The Bell Curve*'s scientific pretensions and underpinnings and been riveted by the question of whether the book's analysis insults or bears witness to what some have described as the nation's democratic, egalitarian legacy, they have more or less greeted its vitriolic reading of the reproductive strategies and practices of African American women with silence. In chapter 6 I query the possible meanings of this silence and their chilling implications and argue that, in effect, such silence keeps in place and at play a set of meanings with respect to black women's bodies that renders Herrnstein and Murray's proposals, as they themselves have claimed they are, both modest and reasonable.

With the discussion of *The Bell Curve* in chapter 6, the attention of the book gravitates toward a corner of the reproductive landscape where border skirmishes in recent years over how genes will signify, culturally—and, thus, over who or what gets to count as fully human—have grown both more inflamed and more perilous. In chapter 7 I linger on this landscape to explore the changing geography of desire and dread that characterizes contemporary responses to new reproductive and genetic innovations, taking up the controversy that erupted in 1993 when it was announced that two researchers from George Washington University, Jerry Hall and Robert Stillman, had cloned seventeen human embryos. Although the experiment itself was considered "unremarkable science," it nevertheless incited a moment of global hyperventilation or "national hysteria," as bioethicist John Fletcher described it. The cloning venture was said to mark both a dangerous turn and a critical juncture in the ongoing showdown between technoscience and humanism. It was also widely condemned for having, if not imperiled, then certainly insulted human difference, singularity, and authenticity or precisely what many commentators seemed to agree distinguishes humans as human and from each other.

What is perhaps predictable but instructive about the border skirmish over cloning is the pervasive fear of "sameness" that was reflected in popular responses to the experiment, particularly given the general cultural intolerance toward "difference" that seems only to have intensified in recent years. Equally as instructive are the collective fantasies of monstrosity that this fear incited and the quick appeal that was made to genetics—as the guarantor of individual originality and authenticity as well as cultural diversity—to keep these monsters at bay. In chapter 7 I suggest that, contrary to popular imaginings, sameness, repetition, and replication are not the issue. As Mary Douglas puts the matter and as we will see repeatedly rehearsed throughout this book, part of the work of institutions is "to bestow sameness or turn the body's shape to their conventions."[19] The issue across discursive arenas is rather how to contain the proliferation of differences or render diversity and difference socially legible, and both of these, I argue, are what geneticizing does. Appealing to genetic essentialism to preserve individual originality and diversity, as many did in the cloning controversy, solves very little in the end. It may ostensibly repair and close to traffic one set of borders that circumscribe the distinctly human, but, as I suggest throughout this final chapter, such an appeal produces its own parade of monstrosities in opening up yet others.

1 / Impaired Sight or Partial Vision? Tracking Reproductive Bodies

I

I want to begin by framing this chapter and collection with a story that Oliver Sacks tells in an article that appeared in the *New Yorker* several years ago. The story is about a man Sacks refers to as Virgil. Virtually blind for forty-five of his fifty years as a result of a series of acute childhood illnesses, Virgil was prompted by his fiancée to visit an ophthalmologist for treatment. He had thick cataracts, writes Sacks, "and was also said to have retinitis pigmentosa, a hereditary condition that slowly but implacably eats away at the retinas."[1] Still, Virgil "could . . . see light and dark, the direction from which light came, and the shadow of a hand moving in front of his eyes."[2] After reviewing Virgil's medical history and examining his eyes, the ophthalmologist determined that both retinas were still functional. In contrast to specialists who "over the years had been unanimous in declining to operate, feeling in all probability [that Virgil] had no useful retinal function,"[3] the doctor recommended that surgery be undertaken to remove the cataracts and to implant a new lens in his right eye. Virgil's mother opposed the operation ("He's fine as he is"), and Virgil himself expressed no strong preference about it either way, but his fiancée was adamant. It was unlikely that Virgil's vision could be fully restored; however, the prognosis for partial recovery was encouraging. As she assessed the situation, partial vision was better than no vision—indeed, in her estimation, Virgil had nothing to lose and might possibly gain a world radically enlarged by seeing.

Virgil underwent the surgery, and the following day, amid the anxious anticipation of those who had gathered around his bed, his bandages were removed. Unlike the redemptive moment staged either at hospital bedsides in countless films or in biblical tales, when scales of both a literal and figurative sort fall from sightless eyes to reveal a world of splendid glory, "the dramatic moment," according to Sacks, "stayed vacant."[4] Virgil's sight had indeed been "restored," which is to say his retina and optic nerve were transmitting impulses, but, by Sacks's account, absolutely nothing happened.

> No cry ("I can see!") burst from Virgil's lips. He seemed to be staring blankly, bewildered, without focussing, at the surgeon, who stood before him, still holding the bandages. Only when the surgeon spoke—saying "Well?"—did a look of recognition cross Virgil's face.[5]

What awaited Virgil once his bandages were removed was not a world of independent, obvious, or self-evident meaning, but a confusing collage of undifferentiated, largely unidentifiable, lines, objects, and colors. Although Virgil could "see," in a literal or physiological sense, what he saw upon his first visual encounter with the world after forty-five years was simply incomprehensible.

> Virgil told me later that in this first moment he had no idea what he was seeing. There was light, there was movement, there was color, all mixed up, all meaningless, a blur. Then out of the blur came a voice that said, "Well?" Then, and only then, he said, did he finally realize that this light and shadow was a face—and, indeed, the face of his surgeon.[6]

Unable to decipher and organize into coherent and recognizable patterns of meaning what he was seeing, and lacking visual memories that would allow him to infer these patterns, Virgil emerged from surgery no longer visually blind, but in a state of mental blindness. The surgery had restored his capacity for sight, but it did not and could not simultaneously restore his capacity to see. Contrary to our working assumptions and everyday experience as sighted creatures, seeing is not only or even primarily a physiological event, an automatic, spontaneous, or mechanical process—something that happens in either a natural or unmediated fashion when we open our eyes to the world. Seeing is rather an act of immense construction, loosely governed by templates that are laid down in the first years of life and performed "seamlessly, effortlessly, and, for the most part, unconsciously, thousands of times a day at a glance."[7] Seeing is a set of learned practices and processes that allow us to organize the visual field and that engage us in producing the world we seem to greet and take in only passively.

Neurologists, psychologists, philosophers, and assorted others who have jockeyed for control of that vast and shifting borderland on which the brain, the eye, and "the self" or cognition, perception, and consciousness are thought to meet will be quick to point out that I have dramatically oversimplified the matter here and, in some sense, of course, I have: the article with which I have chosen to begin appeared in the *New Yorker*, after all, and not in the *New England Journal of Medicine* or any of its more specialized analogues across the disciplines. On top of this, what I have reconstructed is a considerably abbreviated or stripped-down version of Sacks's story, one that leaves out, for example, his discussion of the differentiation that occurs in cerebral development following the early loss of a sense: the cerebral cortex in babies is apparently able to adapt to any form of perception, whereas "the cortex of an early blinded adult such as Virgil has already become highly adapted to organizing perceptions in time and not in space." This makes the switch from a sequential to a visual-spatial mode highly fraught and explains, at least in part, some of Virgil's subsequent difficulty in navigating the world by sight rather than by touch or sound.[8]

Although these details among many others render seeing a rich and complex matter, they nevertheless sit to the side of what I take to be one of the more disruptive and, thus, instructive moments in Sacks's story, Virgil's first moment of visual contact. It is around this moment, clearly, that the story turns, yet in classes where I have used the article, students have tended to resist it, as well as the explanation toward which it encourages us: that our vision is mediated by much more than the eye or trained in the fullest sense of the word; that to be able to "see" the world at all is already to be making sense of it, or making it make the sense it seems a priori to possess. Reaching for an apparently more comforting if also less plausible explanation, many students moved to individualize and pathologize Virgil's confusion. Some students, for example, speculated that Virgil's inability either to grasp the world that offered itself up to him for viewing or, in the months that followed his surgery, to decode and comprehend pictorial and televisual representations of it was the result of undiagnosed medical problems, while others suggested that his confusion was the result of previously unidentified mental ones.

The contorted reasoning that riddles both accounts and reduces blindness to multiple states and levels of masking works to preserve the apparent "givenness" of a well-ordered and transparent world, directly perceived and objectively perceivable. Indeed, both accounts shelter the commonplace assumption, ostensibly more consistent with and thus bolstered by experience—for when has the world ever *not* been in focus?—that seeing simply delivers the world to us, is something for which we are "hardwired" and, thus, a purely natural, hence neutral, activity outside the reach of culture. They shelter the assumption that what we see and how we see are distinct and separable matters. There are things as they "really" are and things as we come to see or interpret them, truth and opinion, reality and representation. Point of view, perspective, and interpretation or the situated and thus circumscribed quality of all vision happen after the fact. They are practices that corrupt, prevent, or occlude sight rather than practices that enable it or, putting the matter more strongly still, constitute its very condition of possibility.

What renders Virgil's first moment of visual contact disruptive is that it disables any easy embrace of the idea of passive vision and, along with this idea, dominant epistemological and ontological assumptions that sustain and are themselves sustained by it. As Donna Haraway, among others, has argued, ways of seeing—of decoding, deciphering, classifying, translating, and interpreting—are not something with which we are simply born, but constitute and are constituted by particular ways of life. They contain and are themselves contained by particular ways of organizing a world (and humans within it) that otherwise seems self-evidently what it is and objectively knowable as such.[9]

By way of example here, consider the ruthless beating of Rodney King by Los Angeles police officers and their subsequent acquittal by a Simi Valley jury notwithstanding a videotape that seemed to provide incontrovertible proof of police brutality. The controversy surrounding the videotape and the contest over what it exposed, what story it told, and what, in the end, it was actually evidence of provide a particularly clear and striking illustration of both Haraway's observations and many of the assumptions about the immediate and unmediated nature of vision that provoked students to personalize and pathologize Virgil's confusions. About the tape and the violence it recorded, Kimberlé Crenshaw and Gary Peller write that "for most people, including most political conservatives, there was no difficulty 'seeing' what [it] represented: old-style, garden-variety racist power exemplified by the Bull Conner/Pretorialike images of heavily armed white security officers beating a defenseless Black man senseless."[10] To the horror and outrage of many, however, this is precisely what the Simi Valley jury ostensibly "failed" to see in determining that the police officers did not employ unreasonable or excessive force in subduing Rodney King but had themselves been put at risk by the body they were beating.[11] Indeed, as the jury came to see the matter, it was not King who was vulnerable, endangered, or threatened, but the presiding officers—all twenty-six of them—and it arrived at this conclusion not by disregarding or dismissing the videotape, but by closely and repeatedly examining it, frame by frame.

So what happened? The tape itself seemed to provide a certain unmediated access to reality. It was presented, and for that matter received, as an unstaged and spontaneous—and therefore disinterested and authentic—record of the sort of terrorism and racist abuse community organizers in Los Angeles had long argued were routinely practiced by members of the city's police force.[12] It captured a moment and in reflecting it back appeared to establish compelling "visual evidence" that many believed could not and finally would not be ignored as previous charges of police brutality had been, so disturbing and ostensibly incriminating was the nightly broadcast spectacle of nightstick meeting skull. However, as attorneys for the officers argued successfully in Simi Valley, what people thought they were seeing and what they were actually seeing, in the end, were two entirely different things. According to the attorneys, although the police appeared to be acting both ruthlessly and recklessly, they were actually performing a series of police-approved restraint techniques to subdue a man they claimed was "bearlike" in strength and immune to pain, in a drug-induced frenzy and resisting arrest.

To make this point, what the defense did, as Crenshaw and Peller explain, was break the video down, frame by frame, into a series of frozen images. Experts on prisoner restraint were then called upon to read these images, to read each still picture, and decipher both King's bodily movements and the baton strikes they incited. According to the experts, no single still alone revealed a stroke that in itself was either excessive or unreasonable;[13] indeed, each discrete stroke, in their view, represented an appropriate, institutionally authorized response to a violent and unyielding suspect, himself "in complete control [of the situation] and direct[ing] all the action."[14] What the defense did, in other words, was anatomize and renarrativize the images, drawing forth from the video an altogether different story from the story it was heard initially to speak. When viewed and (re)interpreted frame by frame, the tape could be and was said to reveal "not incredibly clear evidence of racist police brutality, but . . . , ambiguous slices of time in a tense moment that Rodney King had created for the police."[15]

It is tempting to reject the strategy of close reading that the lawyers for the defense pursued as well as the verdict that resulted and to insist that the clear and powerful evidence the tape appeared to capture was manipulated, misread, misconstrued, and mishandled. This was certainly the impulse of many when the jury handed down its judgment, and there is much about the court proceedings to reinforce the moral indignation that incites it. Without dismissing this impulse, what I want nevertheless to pause over is the assumption that grounds it, the "positivist fantasy," as Robert Gooding-Williams characterizes it,[16] that the meaning of the event is transparent, objectively fixed, and self-evident, that the jury's judgment ignores the clear and obvious facts of the matter or flagrantly denies what "really" happened. This fantasy is but a variation of the one that informed the response of many students to Virgil's inability to decipher the world that confronted him following surgery. Indeed, both share the idea that the visual field is itself somehow neutral, that the world is simply there and can speak for itself in a clear, unmediated fashion. And the point with respect to Virgil's first moment of visual contact, but sharpened by the King example, is that there is and can be no unmediated account, no reading of the tape, or for that matter one's immediate surroundings, that does not depend on point of view or interpretation or a constellation of narratives that frames an otherwise random set of images (colors, lines, and objects) and makes them make sense. Objectivity—that position that itself escapes positioning, that is somehow outside the particulars of time and place, that "represents while escaping representation" and lays claim to a disinterested and thus privileged gaze— is itself only a story "that has lost track of its mediations,"[17] or, in the case of the video, that has lost track of those narratives, racially framed and circumscribed, that "assign the white bodies appearing in the tape the function of holding the fort of civilization against the willful attack of a chaos-bearing wild animal" or lead us to "see" in the repeated stroke of the police baton "old-style, garden-variety racist power."[18]

The contest that took place in the Simi Valley courtroom was, on one level, clearly, a contest over interpretation—over how to situate and read and, thus, how to see the images depicted in the videotape. At the same time and less obviously, this contest over "how" to see was also a contest over conflicting forms and practices of life—in Haraway's terms, particular ways of organizing the world and, specifically, of organizing and ordering racial boundaries, hierarchies, and relations of power—that are embedded in and sustained by, indeed that make possible, particular ways of seeing. The story that the lawyers for the defense told and invited the jurors to read the tape through—to see the tape as telling—both constituted and confirmed a hauntingly familiar world, one in which "black" had come to function in the backlash years of Reagan and Bush as the site and source of urban disorder and social decay, the sign and symbol of a dark, dangerous, and ever-expanding (moral) wilderness, of "imagined excess overtaking, robbing, needing to be . . . taught a good lesson, needing to be put [and kept] in its place."[19] Working racial fears and anxieties and working from other stories and images of black bodies already interpreted and in circulation, lawyers for the defense produced an account of the tape that was consistent with the production of "blackness" within the culture at large, in Congress and the courts and the popular media as well. Their account conjured for the jury what the jury was, in some sense, prepared or predisposed to see—conjured, as Gooding-Williams puts it, "the Negro it was looking to see."[20] It is this cultural resonance (of meaning) that functioned as adhesive, that rendered the defense's version of what "really" happened, its framing of "blackness" and of King, plausible, true to life, indeed, convincing—that made it, in a word, stick.

II

So what does this preamble, these stories of the partial and mediated character of sight, have to do with the panoply of new reproductive and genetic technologies? Each of the chapters in this collection works to decipher and scrutinize, problematize, and, in places, challenge the shifting logic and operation of particular ways of seeing that produce and are themselves produced by contemporary discourse and debate over new and, in the cases of abortion and traditional surrogacy, not-so-new reproductive and genetic techniques—ways of seeing that have, for example, precipitated the reframing of the juridical position of women and redefined who is a subject with legal standing; that have recast the uterus as public space, embryos as public entities, and pregnancy as a state of endangered captivity, refigured the state's interest in prenatal life, and rehabilitated notions of "natural motherhood"; that have brought into play an age-old mythology that in the genetic blueprint might also lie hidden a social blueprint and breathed new life into once-discredited notions that social ills can be traced to genetic errors. Each chapter in this collection, in other words, aims to make visible and thereby demystify some of the lenses through which we peer, that train our sight, that render intelligible, or not, the changing geography of desire and dread that has shaped and in turn been shaped by the radical transformation of reproductive practices and processes. Each essay maps some piece of what are otherwise elaborate and complex conceptual apparatuses that enable us in this last decade of the twentieth century to manage, make sense of, and maintain our bearings in a world in which conventional forms and practices of life, or extant cultural categories, identities, and relations—what is called mother, father, parent, person, and family—are being reassembled and also reinforced, usually at the same time and thus in ways that often render their articulations both strained and confused.

That there is a logic and operation of seeing at work within legal, medical, scientific, and popular discourses, and not one, but multiple, often contradictory and inextricably contextual, ways of seeing that together configure and are configured by the shifting landscape of contemporary reproductive practices and politics is something I take as self-evident. Consider the 1987 surrogacy case of "Baby M." In this case, a New Jersey Superior Court maintained that its task was to found order on a new frontier, produced by science and unsettled by law. This "founding" engaged the court, as we will see, in refiguring "the natural" from forms of relationship and relatedness that do not—indeed, cannot—arise "in nature." How then was this refiguration achieved? What readings, reasonings, and renderings of nature did the court deploy to accommodate practices that otherwise displace it?

What fantasies of reproduction inform its finding that at her birth the child it called "M" had neither mother nor family but was in effect a "technobaby," born of paternal desire and late-twentieth-century ingenuity? What conceptions of parentage and heritage did the court bring to bear to produce an utterly conventional familial arrangement out of what it had originally claimed was a novel reproductive one? And, finally, how were its determinations with respect to what would count as nature themselves naturalized or renarrativized and performed as matters of fact?

Likewise in the 1991 surrogacy case of Anna Johnson, the black woman who gestated, delivered, and sought custody of a white child to whom she bore no genetic link but with whom she claimed to have bonded, what is the structure of reasoning, of seeing, that underwrites and is underwritten by a California court ruling that Johnson was not the "natural, biological, or real mother" of the child to whom she had given birth, but simply a "foster parent," a "surrogate carrier," a "contractual moment" in the constitution of a technologically enabled but, from the court's perspective, otherwise "natural family"? What constellation of assumptions are at play and make plausible the suggestion that it was racial yearning rather than maternal yearning that incited Johnson's claim and, further, that Johnson herself was someone so lost in a dream of whiteness that she failed to see clearly who she was and to whom the white baby she had "hosted" belonged even when the answer had been scientifically established with DNA tests and was, in any event, visibly apparent? For what readings and relations did these tests function as an authorizing text? What recognitions and identities did they not only confirm but also create?

In both of these cases and clearly in a broader, more general sense, as the discussion of the Rodney King trial also suggests, the court functions as a space of reason. By this I mean not that it is, as it purports to be, a neutral site outside of or set apart from social interests and relations, but that it is a space within which reasonings are enacted and recognitions fixed to produce what they also keep intact, particular forms and practices of life, particular formations and relations of power. Notwithstanding their important differences, both of the two surrogacy rulings work in this fashion or work to restablize as a matter of (natural) fact what they also both presuppose and compel into being. Each ruling, in other words, must contain and rehabilitate alternative stories of origins and kinship. And one of the ways both accomplish this is by retelling these stories in a register that renders them variations on an original story, typically, a highly sentimentalized story of heterosexual love, yearning, and procreative desire. The case of Anna Johnson is particularly striking in this regard.[21] Invoking expert medical testimony, the lower-court judge in this case argued, among other things, that maternal bonds of the sort Johnson maintained had developed over the course of her pregnancy—deep and abiding, "instinctual," bonds—were likely to occur only within the sanctity of a proper family unit, among "married mothers with husbands whose babies they carry."[22] "A three parent, two-mom claim," the judge insisted, constitutes "a situation ripe for crazy-making."[23] A child may now have two biological mothers and up to five parents, but only one "mother" will be recognized as the "real" and, thus, "natural" mother and only one monogamous, heterosexual pair will be recognized as forming a real and thus natural family.[24] And the point is that although such recognitions may seem to be simply a matter of common sense, in line with commonly held premises and expectations, something we already know, they are not necessarily obvious, incontrovertible, or particularly self-evident on appeal to a set of biological facts that are, after all, precisely what the courts have been forced to reassemble into some coherent, discursive whole in the wake of technoscientific interventions into reproduction. They are practices of seeing that constitute and are constituted by what have become in the context of new reproductive innovations often rather curious readings and strained reasonings. Linked to and shaped by larger stories, images, fantasies, judgments, desires, and preferences that circulate within the culture, such recognitions organize and authorize, construct and construe, distinguish and determine which forms of life, claims to relationship, and kinds of identities will be sanctioned as natural and which dismissed, as with Anna Johnson, as simply absurd.

When I suggest, then, or claim and insist that there is a logic and operation of seeing at work or multiple, often contradictory, ways of seeing that shape and are shaped by a shifting reproductive landscape, I am referring, among other things but centrally, to the immense and complex acts of construction that are necessarily entailed in keeping intact and viable the world as it self-evidently appears to be—to how, with respect to the legal skirmishes just sketched, new forms and practices of life, new life forms, and the proliferation of interpretive possibility that accompanies them are rhetorically managed and rehabilitated to (re)produce and fortify precisely what they also disrupt: dominant narratives about who or what is called person, parent, mother, family, baby, and fetus. But, setting aside contemporary legal contests for the moment and shifting focus, we can consider what I have been calling a logic and operation of seeing from a somewhat different angle and through a somewhat different lens, or in terms of some familiar, frequently cited biopolitical remappings of social life. We could begin with Nicolas Hartsoeker's late-seventeenth-century claim, for example, that when he first peered down a microscope to examine semen, he saw little preformed men in the head of sperm. This "discovery" confirmed—decisively, in Hartsoeker's estimation—what Aristotle before him had only surmised: that sperm was itself the sole and vital source of generation.[25] Although we might speculate as to what made Hartsoeker's sighting both possible and plausible—and his was only one among several similar sightings—few of us today, I suspect, would find it a particularly credible rendering of what was swimming around at the other end of his imaging device. Still, he and others "saw" it.

No less curious and improbable than Hartsoeker's finding is the "discovery" of eighteenth-century anatomists that "the essential sexual difference"—indeed, the site of difference, apart from genitalia—was rooted in the skeletal structure, the very bones, of Anglo-European men and women and evidenced most obviously in the pronounced discrepancies between pelvis and skull: whereas the cranium of men was said and shown to be larger (so as "to hold the seeds of civilization"), women reigned in the realm of the pelvis (as befit their perceived procreative/social functions).[26] And then there are the studies of nineteenth-century craniologists who shared with anatomists of the preceding century the desire to locate the essential site and source of racial difference *and degeneracy* and who believed they had found evidence of both in the size, shape, and weight of the "African" brain.[27] Add to these the claims of nineteenth-century physicians who argued that women who willingly threw off the product of conception through abortion or contraceptive use infringed upon natural law and would subsequently suffer sterility, derangement, disaster, and ruin. It would be easy, clearly, simply to dismiss each of these well-known, often-recounted moments of biopolitical remapping in the making of the life sciences as simply "bad science," science driven by interest, ideological commitments, or any of a number of more sinister motives even the least paranoid among us could name without effort. More interesting to consider, and for that matter more pressing, is how socially significant differences were (and continue to be) produced under the auspices of disengaged discovery.

"Conscious fraud in science is probably rare," writes Stephen Jay Gould, and the manipulation or fabrication of data that signals it is not obviously evidenced in the investigations of either eighteenth-century anatomists or craniologists of the nineteenth century.[28] Rather, both sets of scientists believed that their studies were free of cultural bias, believed that the body could and did simply speak for itself, believed, finally, in their own objectivity and, thus, their authority to see, hear, and transcribe the body's permanently silent directives—its conditions as well as its constitution. The question is how this transcription, this text of difference or narrative of justification, was achieved, and the task, then, is to decipher its plot—to decipher, on one hand, the cultural work this text performed, while, on the other, tracking the particular constellation of assumptions and presuppositions or, in Gould's language, "a priori conclusions" about the meaning of socially marked differences and their basis that framed, mediated, circumscribed, and were already implicated in what was regarded as "natural," what counted as "evidence," what was observed and, in the end, could appear within the visual field. How did appraisals of bone and analyses of data organize and enforce difference as incapacity or work to produce race and sex as objects of knowledge while in the process codifying a system of classification that positioned both as naturally subordinate? What renders these appraisals plausible, makes them make sense, lends them explanatory power? What world(s) do they contain and construct, assume and (re)inscribe, yet leave unwritten?

From a distance that is historical, epistemological, and probably also psychological, the logic and operation of seeing—the particular configurations of power or particular discursive practices—clearly at work in eighteenth- and nineteenth-century accounts of discovery and difference generating "new ways of interpreting the body [that were also] new ways of representing and constituting social realities"[29] can be easily ascertained and mapped. Less immediately obvious or discernible are the discursive and material practices of seeing that perform the critical cultural work of producing, containing, legitimating, and instantiating meaning in late-twentieth-century North American life. Indeed, the stakes are considerable for firmly distinguishing between what eighteenth- and nineteenth-century sightings "revealed" as "the actual character of things as they are" and what is now "revealed" as such, between accounts of bones and their contemporary, ostensibly uncompromised and more sophisticated, analogues—investigations that look to the organization of the brain, rather than its weight or size, for the biological basis of presumed gender differences or to prenatal hormonal levels for the origins of homosexuality.[30]

But consider, with respect now specifically to new reproductive practices and processes, what a recent special issue of the *Western Journal of Medicine* characterizes as an "important change in outlook" among physicians in the rapidly expanding field of fetal medicine and reproductive genetics. This change in outlook is attributed by the journal's editors to an "improved ability to 'examine' the fetus in utero,"[31] to new instruments of vision or new imaging technologies that enable practitioners to place the contents of "the once opaque womb" under "the light of scientific observation"[32] and thereby clarify their otherwise "cloudy view" of fetal life.[33] "Stripping the veil of mystery from the dark inner sanctum," as fetologist Michael Harrison describes the facility of new visualizing practices, physicians have encountered what Harrison characterizes as "a shy and secretive fetus," "not the passive parasite [they] had imagined," but a "surprisingly active little creature"[34] behaving in a fashion that specialist Frederic Frigoletto suggests resembles three-year-olds at nursery school.[35] With real-time ultrasound imaging, Frigoletto writes, researchers have "developed a composite picture of the fetal state" and will eventually "be able to establish normative behavior for the fetus at various gestational stages." Such imaging, he continues, "will help us identify abnormal fetal development, perhaps early enough to be able to correct the environment to treat the fetus in utero."[36]

"Correct the environment"? Inside these accounts, which I take up at greater length in chapter 2, and similar descriptions routinely proffered by radiologists, obstetricians, and sonographers reading and interpreting for their pregnant patients the otherwise indiscernible snowy imagery produced by the new visualizing technologies, work of all kinds is being performed under the auspices of an ostensibly passive gaze detached from any field of purpose.[37] The fetus is clearly personified, perceived, presented, and produced as a person who has simply been awaiting discovery or awaiting the development of the right optical instruments for its true nature to be fully revealed and apprehended. What troubles these observations, however, or unsettles the story they tell of disengaged discovery, is a small, but hardly minor, detail: the "once opaque womb" has been transparent, public—indeed, open to the public—since at least 1965, when *Life* magazine first published a series of color photographs shot by Swedish photojournalist Lennart Nilsson and titled, "Drama of Life before Birth."[38]

The obvious question that seems then to emerge is, What exactly does the "light of scientific observation" make it possible to see and apprehend today that was not or could not be seen and apprehended three decades ago? Where physicians were once limited by what they could imagine, Nilsson's images notwithstanding, and could "imagine" only "passive parasites" or "inert passengers," new visualizing practices now apparently reveal what are, instead, prenatal toddlers, preborn individuals who have potential medical problems and normative profiles and who, although "dependent on the mother's nutrient supplies," are said to otherwise "enjoy considerable independence in regulating their own development."[39] In precisely what respects do these contemporary sightings and the "new facts of life" they seem to disclose significantly differ from the claims of nineteenth-century physicians who came to regard the fetus as an autonomous, self-determining life form and argued that its "subsequent history after impregnation [was] merely one of development, its attachment merely for nutrition and shelter"?[40] What distinguishes these contemporary sightings from Hartsoeker's discovery when he gazed through the lens of a microscope, his vision extended and enhanced as well, and discerned little preformed men in the head of sperm? If we regard one as "real" and the other as a fantastic abstraction, an invention, apparition, or metaphor at best, how exactly do we determine which is which, which is fact and which a fiction, which a "true" reflection of what is "actually" present and which "mere" representation, a set of condensed arguments, cultural contests, assumptions, and expectations? What translations and omissions, productions and reproductions are entailed in recasting the fetus as a foreign presence that feeds on or off a woman's body into an individual potentially put at risk by that body? What shifts in the categories or relations that constitute fetus, woman, mother, and gestating body does this new sighting, this new form of seeing, require and contain to be not simply plausible but possible?

Substantive distinctions can obviously be drawn between contemporary investigations and sightings and their late-nineteenth- and early-twentieth-century counterparts, and the stakes in drawing them, as I suggested earlier, are for some quite considerable. But when Patrick Steptoe (founding father of in vitro fertilization and thus foremost ventriloquist for reproductive nature) characterizes as "unthinkable" "willingly creating a child to be born into an unnatural situation such as a gay or lesbian relationship"[41] and asserts as a matter of biological fact and in a fashion reminiscent of his nineteenth-century counterparts that the thwarting of women's procreative drive, whether by chance or by choice, is unnatural and will produce "disturbances"[42]—indeed, when fetologists, radiologists, and sonographers describe the fetus in utero as an autonomous, interest-driven life form or, again, in ways that are resonant of those deployed by nineteenth-century physicians in their drive to refigure the maternal/fetal relation and criminalize abortion—such distinctions, however substantive, significant, or ostensibly relevant, seem, in the end and in some important sense, beside the point. To reiterate what has become a commonplace in feminist and cultural studies of science: medical science, the life sciences, and biology occupy a highly political field and remain today, as in earlier historical moments, culturally constituted and constitutive reading practices, socially embedded ways of seeing that operate apart from law but often with its force to regulate and contain what they, of course, also produce—a proliferation of procreative stories and alternative procreative possibilities. As powerful sources of cultural meaning, they establish, reflect, maintain, and enforce the borders of an incessantly fluid status quo—categories, identities, bodies, and relations that count as natural. And, perhaps more to the point, they constitute one among several competing cultural discourses and one among several pivotal cultural sites in the high-stakes struggle over the making of subjects and social realities.[43]

2 / Containing Women:
Reproductive Discourse(s) in the 1980s

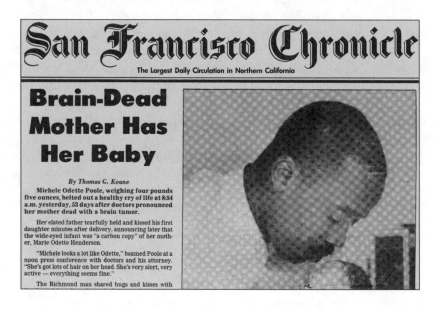

San Francisco Chronicle

The Largest Daily Circulation in Northern California

Brain-Dead Mother Has Her Baby

By Thomas G. Keane

Michele Odette Poole, weighing four pounds five ounces, belted out a healthy cry of life at 8:54 a.m. yesterday, 53 days after doctors pronounced her mother dead with a brain tumor.

Her elated father tearfully held and kissed his first daughter minutes after delivery, announcing later that the wide-eyed infant was "a carbon copy" of her mother, Marie Odette Henderson.

"Michele looks a lot like Odette," beamed Poole at a noon press conference with doctors and his attorney. "She's got lots of hair on her head. She's very alert, very active — everything seems fine."

The Richmond man shared hugs and kisses with

I

"Brain-Dead Mother Has Her Baby"—so read the headline of a major West Coast newspaper in July 1986, when doctors removed an apparently healthy, thirty-two-week-old fetus from the body of Marie Odette Henderson.[1] Henderson had died fifty-three days earlier from a

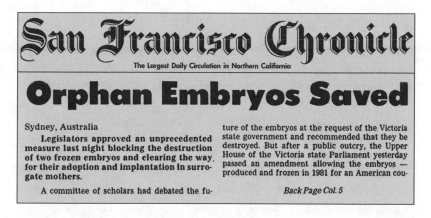

San Francisco Chronicle
The Largest Daily Circulation in Northern California

Orphan Embryos Saved

Sydney, Australia

Legislators approved an unprecedented measure last night blocking the destruction of two frozen embryos and clearing the way for their adoption and implantation in surrogate mothers.

A committee of scholars had debated the fu-

ture of the embryos at the request of the Victoria state government and recommended that they be destroyed. But after a public outcry, the Upper House of the Victoria state Parliament yesterday passed an amendment allowing the embryos — produced and frozen in 1981 for an American cou-

Back Page Col. 5

brain tumor; by court order, her body was kept functioning until the respiratory system of the fetus she carried had sufficiently matured to enable "independent" life. Once matured, the fetus was removed by cesarean section and delivered into the arms of Henderson's fiancé. Shortly thereafter, doctors disconnected the woman from all life support, whereupon she was pronounced dead, again.

Henderson is not the first woman to have been maintained on a mechanical support system until the fetus she carried could survive delivery. In 1983, the "life" of another comatose, legally dead, pregnant woman was similarly prolonged until the twenty-two-week-old fetus she carried had matured.[2] And even as Henderson's doctors in California were disconnecting her respirator, their Georgian counterparts were pumping hormones, oxygen, sugar, protein, and fat through the body of yet another woman in the hopes of rescuing her fetus.[3] As of 1986, there had been at least twelve infants produced in this fashion and, given the generally favorable reception that has greeted their arrival, there is no reason to expect that others will not follow.[4]

Bizarre? Chilling? The stuff of *National Enquirer*, B-grade thrillers, or punk rock lyrics? Consider another headline, appearing in the same West Coast newspaper in October 1984, some twenty months prior to the Henderson event. Reminiscent of those following the release of the American hostages from Iran, this one read, "Orphan Embryos Saved."[5] Orphan embryos saved—embryos we do not usually think of as "orphanable," as independent life forms floating about in the world, as parentless minors, in trouble, on the loose, lost, lonely, abandoned, in need of being saved, "rescued," or adopted. To the degree that we think of them as being "in the world" at all, it is as attached and "embodied"—in a body, part of a body, and a body that is, still, necessarily and exclusively female.

That embryos might be in the world, "parentless" or "detached," "unembodied," and "unembodiable" without dramatic legal—not to mention medical—intervention suggests a dicey situation indeed, and it was into just such a situation that the embryos referred to in the headline had apparently been cast. In vitro grown, "on ice," and awaiting implantation at the Queen Victoria Medical Centre in Melbourne, Australia, these two embryos faced what many considered an unnecessary, not to mention "untimely," thaw when "parents" Mario and Elsa Rios died suddenly in a flying accident. Following their deaths, an intense legal skirmish erupted over disposal of the embryos. Whose property were they, what was their status, the nature of their relationship to each other and their "genetic sponsors," the extent of their claims? Should they be thawed and flushed, used for experimentation, or "put up for adoption"? If "adoptable," were they to be separated or kept together? And once adopted, implanted, and born, did they have rights in the distribution of their "parents'" apparently quite considerable estate?

Various courses of action were being pursued by various interested parties—Michael Rios, the son of Mario Rios by a previous marriage, right-to-life groups in the United States and Australia, as well as potential surrogates from around the globe—when several more announcements were issued regarding the identity and status of the embryos. First, the infertility center at which the embryos were being stored revealed that, technically speaking, the Rios embryos were not in fact orphans at all. They had been conceived with sperm from an anonymous donor and were thus unrelated to Mario Rios genetically; a "biological parent" was indeed alive somewhere, although one clearly uninterested in the many possible ends to which his sperm might have been put. Following this announcement, Carl Wood, head of the "infertility team" at the Melbourne center, disclosed that it was quite likely that the embryos themselves were "duds"—damaged and simply not viable "since [they] had been frozen at a very early period in the development of the freezing technique."[6] None of the embryos frozen at that time, according to Wood, had successfully implanted or developed.[7]

These details had little influence on how the issues continued to be construed and constructed publicly, as the headline "Orphan Embryos

Saved" attests. Against the recommendation of a "committee of scholars," the Rios embryos were "saved" by the Victoria State Parliament
when it passed IVF-related legislation regulating the procedure and
providing, specifically, for the anonymous donation of "orphaned"
embryos to women unable to produce eggs themselves. Presumably,
the two embryos were donated or "adopted"; about what ultimately
became of them, we can only speculate.

Setting aside the particulars of each case for the moment, let us consider again both headlines: "Brain-Dead Mother Has Her Baby," "Orphan Embryos Saved." What makes these headlines make sense? Why
might they seem "sensible" today when only twenty years ago they
would certainly have been preposterous? What is the context, the subtext of utterances that conjoin the banal and the extraordinary in a
temporarily dissonant or disruptive way? What beliefs, assumptions,
and expectations allow them to be coherently rendered, taken seriously, understood as "fact" rather than "fiction"? What is the world
they simultaneously construct and contain? What are the stories they
tell about reproductive possibilities, relations, and relationships in
late-twentieth-century America, and what is the terrain they occupy
and contest in that telling?

Conceptually, both headlines produce a kind of mental astigmatism;
meanings temporarily blur, lose definition, appear distorted, and are
resolvable only with some sort of conceptual retraining or adjustment.
They require us to do conceptually, it seems, what lenses would do op-
tically: refocus, reimage, reintegrate. But just as lenses may enable us
to see the world, they also transform the world we see. And so too
with these headlines. To correct the astigmatism or resolve the various
conceptual distortions they present initially requires a reassembling of
images and familiar categories; however, the ordered, coherent world
we then "retrieve" is one we are also, through this process of reassembling, engaged in constructing. The headlines do not simply present a
world that we passively perceive and assimilate, they also and significantly engage us in the making of one.

Consider again the first headline: "Brain-Dead Mother Has Her
Baby." The coherence of this statement rests, in part, on a very particular understanding of "motherhood," an understanding in which
motherhood is equated with pregnancy and thereby reduced to a physiological function, a biologically rooted, passive—indeed, in this case,
literally mindless—state of being.[8] Within this understanding, mother-

hood is cast as "natural" or "instinctual," a synonym for female, the central aspect of women's social and biological selves, the expression and completion of "female nature." It is something that just "happens," something that is initiated at conception, something that, as a biologically rooted capacity, does not depend upon a woman's consciousness for its development, but develops *as* woman's consciousness if not disturbed or thwarted in the process.

Now, there are certainly other possible understandings of what "motherhood" is and entails. In the United States, conflicting claims and assumptions about its place and meaning have been at the center of many of the most fiercely waged political battles and policy disputes of the past two decades: the struggles, for example, over contraception use, abortion, surrogacy, welfare reform, divorce, child custody, and day care. It is, however, only within this narrow, ideologically biologistic understanding of the term *mother* that the headline itself actually makes sense. Consider an alternative understanding, one that, for example, regards pregnancy as a biosocial experience and motherhood as a historically specific set of social practices, an activity that is socially and politically constructed and conditioned by relations of power, and that differs according to class, race, history, and culture. In this formulation, "being a mother" is not something women "are" by nature, instinct, or destiny, or by virtue of being female or pregnant. Rather, it is something women (among others) do: it is conscious and engaged work in the fullest sense of the word and an activity that is still but need not necessarily be gender specific.

The differences between this account and the first are quite dramatic, resting, as they fundamentally do, upon a distinction between social activities and meanings on the one hand and "biological processes" on the other. Were the latter account a culturally pervasive understanding of the concept "mother," the headline itself would be virtually unintelligible. It is not culturally pervasive, however, and would probably strike a fair number of the population as a somewhat extreme, certainly radical, politically interested formulation, so deeply entrenched is the assumption that motherhood is a (natural) condition, a state of bodily being rather than deliberate activity. It is this assumption—so common as to appear simply part of the "fabric of fact"—that the headline draws upon and reinforces: motherhood is something, it suggests, that simply happens and that can be sustained by mechanical means and a continuous infusion of chemicals even if there is no subject, no agent, to sustain it. The subject that knew herself as Marie Odette Henderson, after all, is dead; *she* is not present, nor for that matter is she represented except as absence or trace. Featured in the picture accompanying the headline is Henderson's fiancé, Derek Poole, cradling the infant over which he sought and won legal custody when Henderson's next of kin authorized doctors to disconnect her respirator. Indeed, to the extent that anyone actually *has* a baby, it is Poole rather than Henderson. In her present state, Henderson is, literally, a receptacle—a quite passive receptacle—for the maintenance of fetal life. She, as Aristotle might have only dreamed, is all biological process, raw reproductive material maintained by extensive mechanical and chemical manipulation. The only sense in which it could be said that *she* is a *mother* who *has* a baby is if her *sheness* is reduced to motherhood is reduced to all biological tissue and process.

Now, there are any number of other ways in which the headline could have been written, and some of these alternative constructions would have proffered a somewhat less sentimental presentation of the Henderson case. The headline might have read, "Thirty-two-Week-Old Fetus Extracted from Corpse"; Eight-Month-Old Fetus Extracted from Dead Woman's Body"; "Deceased Delivered"; "Deceased Maintained, Fetus Successfully Retrieved"; or even "Trapped Fetus Lives." Each alternative rendering offers a more explicit account of the situation, although an account that is also more morbid, disturbing, and potentially destabilizing. What these headlines do that the original does not is foreground the third-party intervention, the hand that reaches into a surgically opened uterus and removes the fetus, the technology that permits the crossing of a hitherto uncrossable border. They make visible precisely those procedures and decisions that the original headline subsumes within the category of biological processes. They denaturalize what the original headline invites the reader to treat as normal—what is more "natural" than mothers having babies? Conversely, what is more "unnatural" than women who try and can't or women who simply won't?

What makes this particular mother having this particular baby newsworthy is that the former is brain-dead; but being brain-dead and having a baby are not necessarily mutually exclusive states when motherhood is considered a physiological "event" that expresses and completes "female nature." "Giving Life after Death"—that is how *Newsweek* ambiguously cast its headline to the story it ran on the

Henderson case. And although it is not clear who is actually "giving life"—the doctors, the courts, or a vast array of biomedical procedures—a perfectly plausible reading of the headline, and one that calms us, suggests it is Henderson, the "mother," particularly if "motherhood" is again understood in the culturally pervasive terms of the original headline. For what motherhood entails, within the sense invoked by the original headline, is commitment, dedication, and self-sacrifice, and what could be a more complete, absolute, or total expression of maternal commitment, self-sacrifice, and dedication than "giving life after death"? Henderson herself, of course, is not a conscious agent in this giving, but then neither are pregnant women more generally. Within the terms assumed by the original headline, they are merely the mediums or physical vessels for new life, not active participants in its creation or maintenance.

II

Throughout this past decade and a half, and particularly during the 1980s, public discourse and debate have been obsessively preoccupied with women and fetuses. The 1980s began, need we remind ourselves, in a flurry of antiabortion, antigay, anti-ERA, profamily, prolife, pro-American rhetoric. According to the story this rhetoric told, the country had grown economically weak, militarily soft, morally decadent, spiritually impoverished, and sexually debauched; newly elected conservatives vowed a "return to basics." This entailed a full-scale assault on affirmative action, civil rights, welfare provisions, and much of the other progressive legislation and judicial action of the previous twenty years.[9] It also entailed a mass-based crusade against liberal abortion and all that the practice marked: teenage sex, nonmarital sex, nonreproductive sex, hedonism, careerism, women's workforce participation, the denigration of "traditional" gender identities, and the dissolution of the nuclear family.[10] Indeed, in the early years of the 1980s, abortion became not only the symbol of the general malaise that was slowly but persistently destroying the social body (as it destroyed the natural-familial-maternal body), but the ideological centerpiece of the New Right's campaign to revitalize the country politically and rehabilitate it morally.

Thus, in April 1981, a Senate Judiciary subcommittee headed by conservative Senators John East and Orrin Hatch began hearings to determine the life status of the fetus. The purpose of these hearings was to bring before Congress the Human Life Statute, or S. 158—a bill that located the beginnings of "actual human life" at conception on the basis of "present-day scientific evidence" and sought to extend Fourteenth Amendment protection to that life, thereby challenging the Supreme Court's 1973 findings in *Roe v. Wade*. The Court declined in *Roe* to make a (formal) determination as to the life status of the fetus. As Justice Blackmun put it, "When those trained in the respective disciplines of medicine, philosophy, and theology are unable to arrive at any consensus, the judiciary, at this point in man's knowledge, is not in a position to speculate as to the answer."[11] The Court nevertheless established "a postnatal condition as a prerequisite for constitutional protection."[12] Maintaining that "the unborn [had] never been recognized in law as persons in the whole sense," Blackmun concluded that, within the language and meaning of the Fourteenth Amendment, the word "person" did not have any possible prenatal application.[13] Were the fetus's "personhood" subsequently confirmed, proven, or somehow "discovered," the Court seemed to imply in *Roe*, its right to life would then be guaranteed specifically by the Fourteenth Amendment, and this was precisely what proponents of S. 158 sought to establish in the context of these hearings: "that the life of each human being begins at conception" and that the Fourteenth Amendment's guarantees extend to all human beings without regard to their gestational stage.

To establish this finding, backers of S. 158 solicited testimony from embryologists, chemists, geneticists, and biologists—in short, prominent members of that community generally regarded as disinterested, beyond reproach, and able to provide, in our age, what philosophers as well as theologians provided in a more distant one: self-knowledge, knowledge of origins, knowledge of the stuff out of which we are made, but knowledge that is rooted in truth—objective, morally neutral, and untainted by the world. Indeed, expert after expert witness testified in support of S. 158, "portraying its thesis as a report from the laboratory," while colleagues and critics alike challenged their authority and expertise as scientists to make factual determinations about the beginnings of human life.[14] According to Leon Rosenberg, head of Yale's genetics department and the only dissenting voice to be included in the initial and most visible round of testimony, such determinations were beyond the purview of science. To Rosenberg's knowledge, raw, scientific data that might be used in defining human life simply did not exist. This claim was echoed by the National Academy of Science when it warned that S. 158 would not stand up to scientific scrutiny, dealing as it did with moral and religious matters or "question[s] to which science [could] provide no answer."[15]

Despite these objections and others, including the charge that S. 158 circumvented avenues provided by the Constitution for reversing Supreme Court interpretations and thus represented an attempt to exercise unconstitutional powers,[16] the Senate Judiciary subcommittee concluded, on the basis of the "evidence" before it, that "science" had indeed "demonstrated" the presence of human life at conception. The fetus emerged from these hearings a "person," but one without constitutional protection and thus vulnerably situated in liberalism's mythic state of nature, where, even for the most clever postnatal entity, life is at best inconvenient and at worst solitary, poor, nasty, brutish, and short.[17]

Although the Human Life Statute and its subsequent incarnations were not ratified, these hearings were quite successful in initiating a process of public redefinition and setting its terms. It is true that the meaning of the Fourteenth Amendment's operative word *person* was not formally broadened to include fetuses. Profoundly discredited, however, was the Supreme Court's interpretation of that meaning, a discrediting accomplished largely by members of that community popularly regarded as trafficking in "truth" and having a corner on "objectivity."[18] Similarly, although efforts to establish a strictly scientific basis for determining fetal personhood were greeted with considerable skepticism, as little more than a dubious political ploy, in the years following these hearings invocations of and appeals to "scientific knowledge," "evidence," and "advances," have become quite commonplace in the dispute over fetal personhood, and not just by those pressing for abortion's recriminalization. Indeed, with these hearings, "science" entered the political mainstream as a reservoir of nonpartisan truths about reproductive relations and has since become perhaps *the* most important ingredient contributing to the transformation of popular perceptions of the fetus.[19]

Initiating the decade of the 1980s, then, are legislative efforts to redefine constitutional language, broaden the meaning of the word *person,* and give concrete reality to the idea of "fetus as person." These legislative efforts have a potent analogue in popular discourse with the appearance of strange and fantastic images of fetuses in bus terminals and public restrooms, as well as on billboards, magazine covers, and the evening news. These images present a prenatal entity with seemingly translucent skin, suspended in empty space or floating free, vulnerable, autonomous, and alone, sucking its thumb in some representations, raising its hands beseechingly in others. A written text usually accompanies such portraits and might pose a question ("Aren't they forgetting someone?"), make an assertion ("Unborn babies are people too"), or issue a call to action ("Stop the killing!"). Now, what this is supposed to be an image of seems obvious, and it does not appear particularly chimerical or implausible until one stops to consider that no fetus (or, for that matter, image) simply floats, alone, in empty public space, unconnected, self-generating, and self-sufficient. Moreover, no fetus (or image) is self-evidently what it is, thus raising the obvious question: What or who exactly is this? Is it the "natural man" of liberalism's mythic past extended to gestation, independent, alone, but threatened? Is it the "rugged individual" of Reagan's mythic present, abandoned by liberal administrations that could not keep their priorities straight? Is it the explorer or spaceman of the mythic future? Or is it Henry Hyde and other members of Congress who have taken to identifying themselves as "postnatal fetuses"—in Hyde's case, a 653-month-old "postnatal fetus"?

All of these allusions bring this image to life early in the decade. Pivotal, however, in giving the "still life" real life, its "own" story, was the 1984 release of *The Silent Scream*, a video production that invited the American public to witness an abortion from the "victim's" point of view. The video "purports to show a medical event, a real-time ultrasound imaging of a twelve-week-old fetus being aborted."[20] What the viewer sees are shadowy, black-and-white images, interpreted and explained by ex-abortionist physician Bernard Nathanson. Nathanson begins the narration by positioning a baby doll next to the shadow he calls a fetus: "The form on the screen, we are told, is the 'living unborn child', another human being indistinguishable from any of us.'"[21] Placid initially, the "movements" of Nathanson's "unborn child" become, by his account, ever more frantic and anguished as the aspiration begins. "Sensing danger," he tells us, it retreats from the aspirator and attempts, in ever more desperate motions, to escape from its sanctuary turned tomb. It struggles violently with its arms and, seconds before it is dismembered and destroyed, throws back its head in what Nathanson characterizes as a "silent scream."

The Silent Scream was made following a study that appeared in 1983 in the *New England Journal of Medicine*, authored by bioethicist Joseph Fletcher and physician Mark Evans.[22] Fletcher and Evans noted that ultrasound imaging of the "fetal form" tended to foster among pregnant women a sense of recognition and identification of the fetus as their own, as something belonging to and dependent upon them alone. Constituting the stuff of maternal bonding, "the fundamental element in the later parent-child bond," such recognition, Fletcher and Evans claimed, was more likely to lead women "to resolve 'ambivalent' pregnancies in favor of the fetus."[23] Within the context of their study—based, significantly, on only two, entirely unrelated, interviews—early ultrasound imaging appeared, to these authors, to encourage fewer abortions and thus to promote pregnancy. According to Rosalind Petchesky, it was this conclusion that apparently captured the imagination of Bernard Nathanson and the National Right-to-Life Committee and precipitated the production of the *The Silent Scream*. The video, Petchesky observes, "was intended to reinforce the 'visual bonding' theory";[24] not only does it enable us to "experience" and view the fetus as though it existed outside the body, already in relationship with the world, it allows and encourages us to treat it as such, as a discrete but vulnerable entity in need of care.

The use of ultrasound for monitoring early fetal development as well as labor has become increasingly regularized in the United States—well over one-third of all pregnant women can expect to undergo the procedure at some point in the course of their pregnancies, and, were health insurers to underwrite its routine use, many speculate that its already widespread application would expand even more. This may account for why a video such as the *The Silent Scream* is "believable," why the fantasy it presents as "medical reality" is so readily accepted as "objective" and "factual" rather than contrived: paraphrasing Petchesky, the live fetal image of the clinic appears simply to have been transported into everyone's living room.[25]

However, also contributing to the credibility or apparent "facticity" of the video, and, more generally, to the transformation of popular perceptions of the fetus, have been extraordinary advances in the area of neonatology—the emergence of new methods of prenatal diagnosis and in utero treatment as well as the development of ever more sophisticated means for maintaining fetal life outside the body at earlier and earlier stages in its development.[26] Not only have these new techniques and treatments made "the fetus more accessible to the world at large, visibly, medically and emotionally,"[27] they appear, in Nathanson's words, to show "beyond reasonable challenge . . . the specifically human quality of its life."[28] Physician Michael R. Harrison puts the issue this way:

> The fetus could not be taken seriously [we might ask by whom] as long as he remained a medical recluse in an opaque womb; and it was not until the last half of this century that the prying eye of the ultrasound (that is, ultrasound visualization) rendered the once opaque womb transparent, stripping the veil of mystery from the dark inner sanctum, and letting the light of scientific observation fall on the shy and secretive fetus. . . . Sonography can accurately delineate normal and abnormal fetal anatomy with astounding detail. It can produce not only static images of the intact fetus, but real-time "live" moving pictures. . . .The sonographic voyeur, spying on the unwary fetus finds him or her a surprisingly active little creature, and not at all the passive parasite we had imagined.[29]

Indeed, as Dr. Frederic Frigoletto, a pioneer on the frontier of fetal therapy, describes it, observing the fetus in utero is "almost like going to a nursery school to watch the behavior of 3-year-olds."[30] No longer a "medical recluse" or a "parasite," the fetus has been grasped as an object of scientific observation and medical manipulation, not to mention anthropomorphic imagination. Thus, although the various new techniques of therapy and repair have not yet made viable the construction of "fetus as person," they have made quite commonplace the construction of "fetus as patient," an entity requiring a separate physician and often a separate legal advocate, or, following Harrison, "an individual with medical problems . . . [who] can not make an appointment and seldom ever complains."[31] Harrison's choice of words and Frigoletto's comparison are instructive. The fetus is neither a "person" nor an "individual" in the strict sense of either word or, as we have seen, for constitutional purposes. However, both descriptions also make clear that the distinction between "patienthood" and "personhood" is not an easy one to maintain, and the ground upon which it rests has been rapidly eroding.[32]

III

If we have witnessed a growing public preoccupation—indeed, obsession—with fetal life over the course of the past decade and a half, no less obsessive has been the popular preoccupation with women. A special report on abortion aired by ABC's *Nightline* framed the matter, and one could say, the decade of the eighties, this way: "With new technologies peering into the womb, women have been forced to peer into their hearts."[33] Although it is hardly novel to present abortion as a conflict between the opposing claims of fetuses and women, the opening statement of *Nightline*'s special report is striking in that it reformulates this opposition and, in so doing, fundamentally transforms it. The conflict it constructs is not between fetuses and women, but rather between "truth" and "desire": on the one side is "truth"—technology, objective observing, the womb as a thing in itself and the site of self-evident but only recently deciphered meanings, the uncovering of knowledge through scientific investigation; on the other side is "desire"—women, self-reflection, the heart as the site of moral (maternal?) meanings, the recovery of knowledge through introspection. Given the traditional ontological and epistemological valorization of the first term of this truth/desire antinomy, a "conflict" in these terms is clearly no conflict at all. It is, at most, a confrontation the outcome of which is foregone: truth must always overcome desire, desire must always give way. Rendered invisible—indeed, irrelevant—by this formulation is some of the dispute's most fiercely contested ground. Rendered derivative and positioned peripherally to their bodies are women.

Just how truly chimerical this antinomy is becomes clear once its first term, *truth*, is situated and contextualized. Technologies are peering, *Nightline*'s report begins, but technologies, we know, do not themselves "peer"; they are instruments and relations that facilitate or obstruct but, above all, construct "peering." Likewise, "peering" is not itself a benign, impartial, disinterested, or disembodied activity, but is both mediated and situated within interpretive frameworks, points of view, sets of purposes. The question, then, is who is peering, what are they looking for and why, with what predispositions, assumptions, expectations, and predilections? Someone (a physician?) is looking and looking for some "thing" (the fetal patient?), for some purpose (diagnostic?), by "consent" or with the cooperation of the woman in whose body the womb is situated.[34]

And then there is the womb itself, the "object" being peered into, and the commonplace knowledge that fetuses, when they hang out, tend to hang out in wombs—this is (still) a condition of being a fetus, popular representations notwithstanding. By peering into a pregnant woman's uterus, one can expect to encounter at least one fetus, perhaps more. So exactly what new mystery has suddenly been unveiled? What is it that the "new technologies" are now "encountering" that "they" weren't, in some sense, already prepared to encounter? What is being "found" that isn't also being looked for? When fetal pioneers Harrison and Frigoletto "peer," they greet, as we have heard them describe their sightings, "shy, secretive," but "surprisingly active little creatures," behaving like three-year-olds at nursery school. Placing the content of the once "opaque womb" "under the light of scientific observation," they have apparently discovered thirty-six-month-old prenatal toddlers. When Representative Henry Hyde, among other staunch opponents of abortion, turns his gaze to the human world he sees "postnatal fetuses"; when "science" turns an "impartial" eye to the content of the uterus, it now sees "prenatal toddlers." The gaze of Hyde is generally recognized as "interested"; the gaze of science, disinterested. On close inspection, what really distinguishes them?

Situated in opposition to the supposedly unsituated gaze of technology is the second term of the antimony, the truly situated gaze of women, directed not toward the uterus, but toward the heart and the heart as it exists, not in some physiological sense, of course, but metaphorically. "Heart" has its etymological origins in the Greek term *kardian* or *cura*, indicating care or concern, and although its metaphorical associations in the West have varied historically, it has enjoyed a consistent identification as the decisive center of things, the source of multiple truths, the site of moral sensibilities, moral conscience, and even unwritten law.[35] Located within the heart or buried in its depths is a particular kind of knowledge of life's interiors and rhythms or things primal, vital, and sacred—a knowledge that is clearly available to all, but traditionally considered more fully and easily ascertained by women. Indeed, in things of the heart both moral and affectional women have traditionally been regarded as the more literate gender, by virtue of their generative capabilities and their intimate, "primordial" relation to the production and reproduction of life.

Especially interesting, therefore, is *Nightline*'s counterposing of the uterus and heart, given that women's "special" ability to read the heart and coherently render its teachings has conventionally been linked to their uteruses, their ability to create life and sustain it. If women must be "forced" to peer into their hearts, forced to do what once took place "naturally," something has ruptured an organic system of communication, of "knowing" and "doing"; something is clearly awry and that "something" appears to be legalized abortion. Liberalized abortion is commonly depicted within popular discourse and debate as having rendered women, if not dyslexic, then illiterate in affairs of the heart—(unnaturally) uncaring and selfish as well as emotionally and physically hostile to the unborn.[36] In this respect, "peering" technologies function as remedial aids. By exposing the interior life of the pregnant uterus, they enable women to reintegrate "knowing" and "doing" (through visual identification and bonding) or once again to "read" all that is believed to be inscribed on their hearts and act accordingly.

Women's alleged "illiteracy" in matters of the heart has been the focus of much anxious public attention. Despite their obvious benefits, technological developments such as in utero therapies and sonography have been deployed to expose its scandalous extent and thus to perpetuate "the most deadly anti-woman bias of them all, namely, that unless women are carefully controlled, they will kill their own progeny."[37] The images, not to mention the rhetoric, have been powerful and, on some level, clearly persuasive. In April 1982, for example, former President Reagan attributed the then severe unemployment rate to the large number of women entering the workforce.[38] Several months later, "profamily" activists claimed their first victory with the defeat of the Equal Rights Amendment. Underpinning Reagan's otherwise forgettable reading of the troubled economy and at the center of anti-ERA ideology sat the assumption that a woman's essential identity could be fully realized only in the home, as housewife and mother. By seeking paid work outside the family, "follow[ing] the siren call of women's liberation . . . and competing in the labor force for scarce available jobs," women were said to be not only jeopardizing the family's stability (as well as the nation's), but denying their natural, God-given destiny to bear children and rear them.[39] Just how inescapably perverse or unnatural women's participation in the workforce is was graphically established, according to prolife forces, by the horrifying costs such participation exacted yearly: quite contrary to their "innate" maternal drives, women were aborting their unborn. Just as animals kill their offspring when they are disturbed or in some way confused, so too were women killing theirs, in "restless agitation against a natural order."[40]

"Hard" evidence could hardly be marshaled to support these clearly dubious claims. However, innuendo and insinuation in the context of what were largely successful efforts to breathe real life into the still life of the fetal form have proved every bit as effective in providing a convincing and compelling portrait of women as out of control and maladjusted, not to mention miserable, agitating against nature, and thus unable to "read" its directives accurately. Consider, in this regard, the development of fetal protection statutes. In 1982, the same year the president told American women to go home, a small group of obstetricians and geneticists declared that "medicine [was] far enough along for them to start treating fetuses as patients."[41] With this declaration came the rapid expansion of efforts not only to treat the "fetal patient" but to protect it from potential abuse or neglect. Juvenile courts subsequently began to assume jurisdiction over the content of pregnant women's wombs and right-to-life efforts to rescue fetuses through forced medical intervention or incarceration of the women carrying them were intensified and highly publicized. Increasingly subject to legal scrutiny and criminal prosecution were pregnant women who smoke, drank, had sex, ingested legal as well as illicit drugs, refused major surgery (for example, cesareans), failed to follow the advice or instructions of their physicians, failed to obtain adequate prenatal care, worked or lived in proximity to teratogenic substances, or engaged in any range of activities deemed "reckless" and potentially detrimental to fetal life.[42]

Statutes currently invoked to monitor or bring under critical scrutiny the conduct of pregnant women were originally designed to protect pregnant women, to provide criminal sanctions against assailants in cases where assault and battery resulted in the death of a fetus.[43] Expanded to reflect new prescriptions for fetal health and vigorously lobbied for by antiabortion organizations, however, the focus of these statutes has shifted to reflect a substantially different agenda. Primarily concerned not with the harm done *to* women but with the harm done *by* them, these statutes now render the former "victim" a potential assailant (or aborter).[44] Depicting a woman and the fetus she carries as two separate, adversarily related individuals—one a potential killer, the other innately innocent—they engender and promote the notion that, whereas women once nurtured their unborn, they now regularly abuse or neglect them and cannot be trusted not to. Where gestation was itself once the most natural of processes, it has now become treacherous. Additionally reinscribed with these statutes is an assumption as old as it has been intractable, that women are merely vessels, "containers" that can be "opened" in the name of fetal health even if such intervention places their own lives and health at stake.[45]

That such statutes both entail and lend legitimacy to the drastic abridgment of such fundamental rights as privacy and bodily integrity seems obvious: the American legal system has traditionally refused "to recognize the right of anyone—born or unborn—to appropriate the body of another for his or her own use."[46] However, in gendered legal discourse, the female body has rarely been considered a "body" in some general, unmarked sense; to the contrary, the American legal system has traditionally subsumed the female body to the maternal body.[47] Now, where gestation is considered the natural fact of female bodies and the essential core of women's identity, where all women are regarded as "mothers," actual or potential, questions of appropriation are largely irrelevant: a body realizing its destiny can hardly be regarded as a body under siege, a body "appropriated."[48] When such questions do become relevant, therefore, as in the case of fetal protection statutes, they are readily configured as a problem of deviance—of reckless conduct or instincts gone awry. Indeed, that appropriation becomes a question at all reveals a tear in the fabric of fact and a fracturing of the core of women's identity. Fetal protection statutes, then, mend and solder. They reassert the "voice of the natural" where this voice has been muted or silenced and thereby function, perhaps most importantly, as an indictment. Inasmuch as it is through women that this voice has traditionally spoken, fetal protection statutes imply by their mere existence that women have lost heart or touch with the deepest source of their identity and thus become not only dysfunctional but potentially dangerous.

But fetal protection statutes tell only one story among many. If these statutes conjure an image of women stung with a certain Dionysian madness, that image comes to be mirrored and reinforced early in the 1980s by another, ostensibly more forgiving, one: women undergoing abortions only to emerge from their "madness" to a knowledge of the unmistakable horror of what they have done and become.[49] Early in the decade, there "emerges" a "condition" from which it is said an ever-increasing number of women are suffering—a condition that comes to be known as postabortion stress syndrome. By the decade's end, so pervasive will this "condition" appear to have become that Surgeon General C. Everett Koop will recommend committing up to $100 million for its research[50]—a move that mystifies by medicalizing what seems clearly a "discourse-generated" malady, the spread of which is attributable less to the recovery of lost identity than to the alleged "discoveries" of peering technologies, the public proliferation of arresting representations of fetal life, and the equally arresting representations of women taking that life capriciously, casually, and selfishly.

Postabortion stress syndrome narrates the potentially severe physical, psychological, chronic, and debilitating consequences of women's seduction and debauchery by abortion providers, the media, and feminism. It tells a story of subversion, moral laxity or turpitude, and self-mutilation, of women losing a sense of their nature and place, and of their subsequent victimization. But it is also a story of redemption, for what fetal protection statutes achieve through law, postabortion stress syndrome rights through female suffering: "nature" ultimately reasserts itself, through conscience and "absence." Consider a few of the syndrome's vast range of indications: guilt, remorse, despair, unfulfillment, withdrawal, helplessness, decreased work capacity, diminished powers of reason, anger and rage, seizures, loss of interest in sex, intense interest in babies, thwarted maternal instincts, residual "motherliness," self-destructive behavior, suicidal impulses, hostility, and child abuse.[51] Clearly reinscribed here as "health" are fairly conventional codings of women's bodies and lives. But beyond a necessarily inferential account of both the disruption and the restoration of some sort of natural order, what postabortion stress syndrome seems most importantly to provide are reassurance and consolation. Indeed, this may explain why it has so captured the public imagination and the imagination of certain public health officials: exposed in the absence of something to be mothered are maternal instincts, or, in Koop's words, the longings and aspirations of "motherliness"; motherhood is reiterated as women's "true" desire and interest as well as innate need.

Embellishing this picture and embroidering its tragic qualities is the "emergence" of yet another "condition" presented as having already reached frightening proportions by the time it enters popular culture and consciousness midway through the decade: the "epidemic" of infertility. To the images of women killing for reasons of convenience, abusing their "prenatal toddlers" through reckless conduct and neglect, and suffering inconsolably from having "stomped out" life only to realize its "true" nature and theirs, the recent discourse on infertility adds still other images: to the socially deviant and the psychologically deranged, this discourse conjoins the biologically deficient. Each is a face of women's agitation against the natural order, but the special contribution of the infertility discourse lies in its provision of "evidence," scientific evidence, that the ultimate goal of womanhood is motherhood, that who and what women are is fundamentally and inalterably rooted in their reproductive capacity. If there is any doubt about what women should find upon peering into their hearts, this discourse assuages them.

Profiled in the popular press are accounts of women who believed they could "have it all," who "followed the siren call of women's liberation" and, by their own account, "lost all [their] womanness" in the process.[52] Unable to procreate and finding themselves driven by what fertility specialists characterize and treat as an innate need to do so, these women have been reduced to desperate caricatures of their former self-assured selves, struggling with feelings of inadequacy and failure.[53] Also prevalent among these women are feelings of betrayal, guilt, and remorse, for what the popular press makes unmistakably clear is that the present "epidemic" of infertility is largely the result of "lifestyle." According to *Time* magazine, for example, primarily responsible for the "epidemic" are individual choices and attitudes: delayed childbearing; liberalized and pluralized sexual behavior; multiple abortions; pelvic inflammatory disease; sexually transmitted diseases; strenuous athletic activity, such as dancing, jogging, and distance running; and high-stress corporate/professional employment.[54] Echoing Aristotle and Hippocrates, *Time*'s message is not particularly subtle: women's loss of biological function is linked to their denial of this function through the pursuit of nontraditional career paths and other activities. The natural expression or ultimate goals of female instincts are marriage, motherhood, and home; clearly unnatural and even "dangerous" are abortion, delayed childbearing, nonprocreative sex, and women's workforce participation. Resurrecting the adage "Anatomy is destiny," and giving it renewed force, Patrick Steptoe, "father" of the first in vitro conceived or test-tube baby, frames the matter this way: "It is a fact that there is a biological drive to reproduce. Women who deny this drive, or in whom it is frustrated, show disturbances in other ways."[55]

What *Time* and other popular newsmagazines fail to report are precisely those details that expose the apparently seamless and self-evident reality of infertility as a contestable composition of specific and predictable interests. For example, contrary to its popular presentation as a problem that overwhelmingly afflicts white, affluent, highly educated women, the incidence of infertility is actually higher among the nonwhite and poorly educated. Black women are one and a half times more likely to be infertile than are their white counterparts, but it is not black women whom specialists seek to save from their own nonfunctional bodies or to assist in fulfilling their biological destinies.[56] When *Life* magazine chooses to feature the issue of infertility, along with the various new technologies that have been developed to "treat" it, on its cover is situated not a black baby or a brown one, but a pink, blue-eyed toddler.[57] What world is being held in place, however precariously, by the development and use of these new technologies is hardly a mystery. Both text and subtext are straightforward: white women want babies but cannot have them, and black and other "minority" women, coded as "breeders" (and welfare dependents) within American society, are having babies "they" cannot take care of and whom "we" do not want.[58]

Minus its deeply conservative pronatalist and racist agenda, infertility thus features a demographic profile considerably different from that suggested by popular discourse. But also brought into sharp relief when this agenda is set aside is a collection of "causes" radically more disturbing than "lifestyle" trends. Although infertility is generally rendered a problem that afflicts only women in significant numbers, it is the case that men are as likely as women to be infertile, and that the incidence of infertility for both is attributable to a diverse combination of social and iatrogenic factors: environmental pollution, exposure to hazardous toxins in the workplace, and unsafe working conditions in addition to inadequate health care, misdiagnosis of disease, and sterilization abuse. Although delayed childbearing contributes to low fertility rates, it is hardly the only or even primary ingredient generating this "epidemic."

Finally, as for the "epidemic" itself, the actual rate of infertility in the United States has remained relatively constant over the past two decades.[59] What has changed is the expansion of possibilities for treatment, at least so far as women are concerned. Within the past decade and a half, a range of new technological options have been developed that allow women to "overcome" what fertility specialist Carl Wood describes as "nature's defects."[60] Although still experimental and of disputed effectiveness, these techniques have nevertheless been promoted aggressively since their introduction, and much about the sudden appearance of an "epidemic" seems clearly related to their marketing, not only to the involuntarily childless but to funding and regulatory communities as well.

What each of these accounts offers is the beginning of an alternative reading of infertility that challenges its construction and representation within popular culture not only as a "disease" primarily afflicting affluent, highly educated, married white females, but as evidence of a disruption in the natural order of things largely attributable to female deviance. Seen from other angles, infertility cuts a considerably different form. To the extent that it is a problem, that problem is configured by racism, corporate greed, and the effects of socially stratified health care provisions. To the extent that it contains a story, that story joins others in rehearsing the social and physiological ravages of late capitalism. However, through its incorporation into the political-medical discourse on the dangers of denatured women and the disfigured condition of motherhood in a postliberation era, most of the important details of infertility's causes and victims are totally eclipsed. Within the constraints of this discourse and juxtaposed with another of the decade's dominant images, free-floating or dismembered fetuses, infertility functions as a condensed symbol of the consequences of "womanhood" not kept to its natural place.

IV

In February 1989, "after consulting experts in fields ranging from demography to industrial design to medicine to interstellar travel," *Life* magazine offered its readers a tour of life in the twenty-first century titled "Visions of Tomorrow." Dividing the journey into three phases— self, society, and planet—*Life's* cover story opens with a fourteen-inch, two-page glossy photo of a disembodied uterus captioned "MOTHERS OF INVENTION: New Ways to Begin Life." Situated on a steel table, under operating-room lights, with tubes extending out from both sides carrying saline solution to the implanted embryo, the out-of-body uterus is part of a series of experiments on fertility conducted by a team of Italian physicians in 1986. Although subsequently halted on ethical grounds, their research, *Life* tells us, "is expected to be resumed" and to culminate, as the photograph itself suggests, in the production of an artificial womb or placenta. The text continues, "By the

late 21st century, childbirth may not involve carrying [embryos or fetuses to term] at all—just an occasional visit to an incubator not so
different from the one shown at left. There, the fetus will be gestating
in an artificial uterus under conditions simulated to re-create the
mother's breathing patterns, her laughter and even her moments of
emotional stress."[61]

The incubator to which this text refers is not, strictly speaking, an
artificial apparatus replicating the environment of the womb; it is an
impregnated uterus, the womb itself, excised from a body and me-
chanically maintained. We could call it an "incubator," a model of
things to come, as *Life* does, but why then would we call Marie Odette
Henderson (the "brain-dead mother [who had] her baby") "mother"?
What distinguishes the uterus on the steel table from the legally dead
pregnant woman who was maintained by a life-support system until
the fetus she carried had sufficiently matured, her "maternal contribution" simulated by means of a gently rocking bed, music, and the
voices of nurses?[62] Indeed, why is the former declared by some to be
ethically monstrous, dangerous, or threatening, and the latter presented as an exquisite moment in the history of maternal self-sacrifice?
What exactly is the difference between a disembodied uterus gestating
and an embodied uterus when the body that contains it is dead? Both
are "incubators," but about each a dramatically different story is told.
Life's rendering of reproduction is situated in some distant future and
is about bold new beginnings, mastery over the treacherous incon-
stancy of nature, and fundamental reconstitution of the human world.
According to the text accompanying the photograph, "It will demand
as much new thinking in religious and moral terms as it will in medical."[63] But *Life*'s rendering is also about the needs of the infertile, the
unborn, and the prematurely born—it is partly in response to these
sets of interests that this new technology is being developed. By contrast, the story told through Henderson is of things lost or slipping
away, not simply a life, but a world in which mothers are mothers no
matter what. Marie Henderson, dead, is counterpoint to the decade's
discourse on women, the mirror opposite of her living counterpart
who callously takes or abuses life. In the story told through Henderson, the woman dies, but fetus and mother survive. Nature prevails—
mother nature, the nature of mothers—even as nature (death) is
overcome.

Now, the interesting thing about these two stories is that each contains and constructs the other. The world held in place by Henderson as brain-dead mother, the world of conventional gender meanings and identities, is precisely the world the new technologies of reproduction destabilize; paradoxically, the world these new technologies destabilize is also reinscribed by their ostensible purpose and use as well as by the stories they appear to tell. What, after all, currently legitimates the development of reproductive technologies? They are said to help women realize their maternal nature, their innate need to mother. And what happens to women if this need is denied or frustrated? According to fertility specialist Patrick Steptoe, "they show disturbances." Yet, even as "maternal nature" is asserted, the certainty of what it is and the ability to render it coherently are profoundly shaken. Is Henderson "mother," incubator, or "prototype"? Or consider "surrogate motherhood," where the desire to conserve "nature" and "tradition" results in their utter disruption. As ethicist Arthur Caplan notes about the "Baby M" trial, "This case chips away at our certainty of understanding our concept of mother. It's socially and culturally disturbing. It takes away a reference point."[64] Is it really any wonder that courts and legislatures across the land moved so quickly to outlaw the procedure and fertility specialists began to see in the development of the artificial uterus a viable, ethically preferable alternative?[65]

There are, of course, still other conceptual incoherencies and cultural disturbances generated by the application of new reproductive technologies and techniques. There are free-floating fetuses said to be in need of protection from their "natural carriers," "more helpless . . . than the tenant farmer or mental patient,"[66] and somehow safer outside the womb than in it. There are prenatal toddlers and postnatal fetuses, embryos on ice and "orphaned," frozen embryos apparently so numerous now as to constitute a "national population," and frozen embryos at the center of an increasing number of intense legal skirmishes prompted by divorce. Are these embryos "joint property or offspring," asked a recent headline regarding a particularly acrimonious case in Tennessee. "He" maintains they are joint property and does not want his wife "to attempt to bear his child" using the embryos after they are divorced. As he sees it, he has "an absolute right to decide whether or not he will become a parent."[67] She contends that they are living things, "pre-born children," offspring. Indeed, as she sees it, she has more rights "as the mother"[68] and seeks "to rescue her babies from the concentration camp of the freezer"—where, it must be remembered, she herself interned them.[69] According to her lawyer, hers "is the yearning of a woman to be a mother"[70]—except, of course, "natural motherhood" presupposes a world of male prerogative, one in which his rights are, as he claims, absolute.

Here, as in cases sketched elsewhere in this chapter and book, invocations of natural rights and relations, maternal yearnings, and paternal prerogatives all draw upon, conjure, and attempt to reconsolidate a pregiven, properly ordered world of fixed meanings and identities. Indeed, such invocations aim to recover and stabilize what is perceived as having become temporarily decentered, and in this they are clearly and blatently reactionary. However, in their move to restabilize, invocations of the natural also contain a certain political possibility: contradictions that cannot be resolved or suppressed, a fracture in the dominant discourse that suggests a dramatic weakening of its strength, a disruption in privileged narratives that render them highly vulnerable to contestation. At such moments, a space opens for the entry of new voices and political alliances as well as new interpretations, understandings, and conceptualizations of practices that are a site of social conflict but whose meanings and organization are by no means given.

It is difficult to see in the regressive and reactionary character of the 1980s discourse on reproduction anything remotely resembling alternative, liberatory political possibilities. Throughout much of the decade, those of liberal, left, and feminist political commitments together scrambled merely to defend "women's rights" against a continuous onslaught of legislative, judicial, and medical incursions and were forced, moreover, toward a range of narrowly construed and often confused political responses and settlements. Within the terms, boundaries, categories, and codings of the decade's discourse on reproduction, political possibility appeared and was drastically cirumscribed. But read differently, read symptomatically, the sheer and concentrated attention directed throughout the decade toward disciplining and managing women's bodies and lives—the fierce and frantic iteration of conventional meanings and identities in the context of technologies and techniques that render them virtually unintelligible—signals, among other things, the profound instability and vulnerability of privileged narratives about who and what "we" are. What looks like the narrowing of possibilities from one angle betokens their presence and proliferation from another.

Contained in the disruption of conventional meanings and identities and their particular vulnerability to contestation are numerous possible political openings—multiple points of resistance as well as projects of reconstruction. Naming and seizing these possibilities, however, requires imagination, a new political idiom, as well as a certain courage—to eschew a lingering attachment to things "natural" and "foundational" and to jettison the essentialism clung to by all extant participants and opponents of the repro-tech drama. It requires the courage to take seriously the socially and technologically produced opportunity to invent ourselves consciously and deliberately, and in this to develop the practical, political implications of the philosophical claim that "we" are only and always what we make.

3 / Fetal Exposures:
Abortion Politics and the Optics of Allusion

I

Over the course of the past decade, the grammar and culture of abortion have been profoundly refigured. Although a variety of factors have converged to produce this refiguration, among the most pivotal has been the increased public presence of the fetus. The circulation of fetal images by antiabortion forces, the routine use of ultrasound in monitoring pregnancy and labor, and the development of widely publicized and culturally valorized medical techniques in the area of fetal therapy and repair have together worked to shift the terms in which abortion is now framed, understood, experienced, and spoken, even by those who champion "choice."

In this essay, through a close reading of a 1991 video titled *S'Aline's Solution*, I explore some of the ways in which the public presence of the free-floating fetal form has fundamentally reshaped both the perceptions and practices that constitute abortion and the parameters of contemporary debate. Produced and directed by video artist Aline Mare, this nine-minute video offers an account of one woman's struggle to come to terms with an aborted pregnancy. It depicts a moment of refusal and casts about in the longing and loss that follow that moment in search of a certain redemption.

The video speaks, as we shall see, in a distinctly post-1980s idiom with respect to abortion, deploying many of the same visual and rhetorical strategies used by prolife activists throughout the past decade to tell its story of loss, even as it also claims to affirm in that telling a "prochoice" position. Thus, for example, the video's primary mode of visual argumentation is rooted in the authoritative power of science and medicine. In this respect, the piece is clearly reminiscent of *The Silent Scream*, a 1984 National Right-to-Life Committee production that claims to show in real time, through ultrasound, an abortion from the point of view of a twelve-week-old fetus. Indeed, like *The Silent Scream, S'Aline's Solution* appears to present a medical event, or at least the biological facts of the matter that is abortion, beginning with the penetration and occupation of the "natural body." In much the same way as any of the many PBS or National Geographic specials on the wondrous workings of the human body might begin—by bringing present but hidden processes to light—the video extends our vision, technologically, beyond the everyday apparent through the use of prosthetic imaging devices: we enter a body and subsequently witness what appears to be the initiation of a second-trimester abortion, a saline abortion. In succeeding frames, we encounter the fetus in various stages of development and, in the end, become spectators to its final expulsion. The question is whether the story of struggle this video sets out to tell can be heard in the terms in which it is told. Can what are, in effect, prolife representations, meanings, and practices be (re)-appropriated and oppositionally inflected to tell precisely the kind of story their deployment has otherwise worked to silence? What social, historical, cultural, and ideological terrain does the video's narrative ultimately contain and contest as well as inhabit and produce? In what respects does the "prochoice" stance it claims and articulates make sense as such and what does the "sense" it "makes" in the end tell us about the contemporary grammar and culture of abortion?

II

With the video's opening sequence, we travel up a long, canal-like aperture at a slow and deliberate pace, indeed, a pace that accentuates the drama of our presence in, and encounter with, a region only recently opened for public tours—the irreducibly natural, incontestably given, seemingly "real" body, the body in all of its irreducible, functional glory. And we travel, at least initially, without being told either where we are or where we are going. Nor do we know in whose body, and by whose sponsorship, this high-tech expedition is taking place. That we are sponsored we can be certain, for one never simply or casually crashes these borders, traverses the boundaries between inside and out, penetrates and occupies biospace, on a lark. Any expedition upon which we might set out will be authorized and highly supervised—we will need an interpreter, in any event, someone or some way to decipher what it is we are and will be seeing.

The video's title works, to some extent, to orient us, and so too its audio, a persistent bass drone that is reminiscent of Hitchcock—foreboding, suspenseful, anxiety inducing. Together, they establish a climate of expectation; indeed, both call into play a series of assumptions that initiate the narrative and allow this opening image to mean. Clearly, we are entering a particular social text, even as we appear only to be entering a self-evidently natural or biological one. Still, we are confidently situated within the narrative only with the next series of images and the voice-over that frames them. These images seem to establish beyond doubt in whose body this excursion of discovery has been undertaken, while the voice-over suggests for what purposes: "I choose, I chose, I have chosen." Each utterance is set off by a woman's face, pressed against glass, wet and distorted, and sends us tripping down the bioscape in the general vicinity of a reproductive tract. Here, we witness three discrete moments in the reproductive cycle: a follicle hosting a ripe ovum; the ovum itself surrounded by nutritive cells and water; and the fimbria, or outermost fringe of the fallopian tube, "brushing" the swollen follicle shortly before ovulation. With the assertion of a principle that has grounded feminist demands for reproductive autonomy for more than a century but is most commonly associated with mainstream liberal struggles of the past two decades around abortion rights, this first sequence of images is given closure: "I choose, I chose, I have chosen"; "My body, my choice."

The next segment of the video moves to instantiate "choice," to enact what is an abstract value or claim through the staging of a second-trimester abortion—a saline abortion. Rock salt falls from a hand situated at the top of the screen in one frame, its direction reversed in the next. This is choice reconfigured in the wake of the reproductive discourse of the 1980s, choice that knows and speaks itself, indeed, is permitted to speak publicly, only in the idiom of ambivalence, apprehension, and psychological perplexity. The persistent bass drone

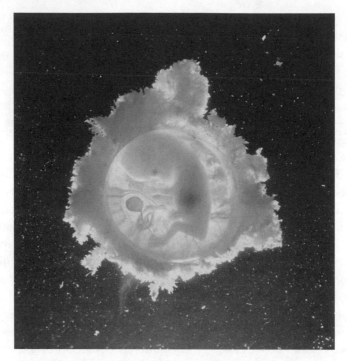

Copyright Lennart Nilsson. From A Child Is Born *(Dell Publishing Company, 1990), used by permission.*

intensifies, as does the sound of running water. In the event that we do not know what a saline abortion is or what it entails, a running text at the bottom of the screen joins with the visual text to provide us with the technical details. In fact, written text is deployed twice in this segment of the video; it serves not only to bracket a montage of images of otherwise discrete bodily processes but to instruct us as well in their reading, even though we have been pursuing this moment since the video's opening sequence. This is its moment of truth, or at least the moment when we will see revealed the truth of the matter that is abortion.

The first written text we encounter, then, initiates the abortion sequence: "saline solution: 200 milligrams of salt and water injected into the uterus causing violent contractions within minutes." The second written text closes it: "sodium chloride . . . salt preserver . . . salt destroyer." Between these two moments, we find ourselves positioned once again within the body, spectators to an apparent real-time abortion from what we are encouraged to infer is the unmediated view of the "victim." We see first a grainy, undulating mass of blue liquid followed by the eruption of bodily fluids: the discharge of a thick, white substance through porous tissue; muscle in spasm; the flow of what looks to be the same white substance, the saline solution, through a narrow, tunnel-like opening; and then, once again, the mass of blue liquid. Although these images are not in themselves either violent or traumatic, their organization, rapid pace of presentation, and curiously alien character foster the impression that something both violent and traumatic, alien and distinctly "unnatural," has just taken place. This impression is encouraged by both of the written texts—we are prepared to see violent contractions and salt destroying—as well as by the posture of the woman in whose body we imagine this abortion to be taking place, the same woman who appeared earlier behind glass. She is now lying on her back, eyes pinched closed, writhing in what seems to be a pain-induced dream state. Rock salt falls on her face like snow while mournful groans grow in pitch and overcome the droning music. The camera closes in on her features and fixes our gaze in a studied, lingering look typically reserved for lovers. The screen then goes blank.

The uneasy intimacy into which we have been drawn is broken by the sound of a child's laughter and the image of an eighteen-week-old fetus floating before us, intact and presumably in utero. "In the face of th[is] portrait of fetal tranquility, the spectre of bodily dismemberment strikes an especially powerful chord";[1] indeed, we cannot help but wonder whether this is the fetus whose death it is we have just seen initiated. "Sh, baby," a voice coos, "baby sh."

In this third and last segment of the video, we are transported into the world of the imaginary—a world of tortured desire and festering loss, of fractured and distorted meanings. And yet it is also a world not easily distinguished from the one produced in and through contemporary medical-scientific discourse under the sign of the real, or the one occupied by prolife advocates in public discourse and debate over the meaning of abortion. Our loss of bearings is immediate and profound. There are the images themselves: these are the work of Swedish photojournalist Lennart Nilsson and are appropriated—as is all of the video's bioscape imagery—from *Miracle of Life*, a documentary originally aired on the PBS series *Nova*. Under the auspices of science, this award-winning documentary purports to unveil not only the mysteries

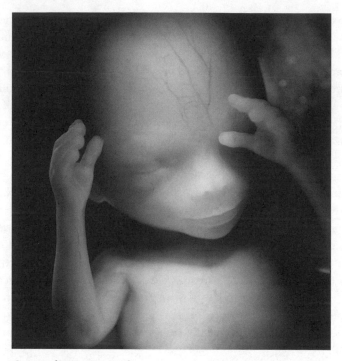

Copyright Lennart Nilsson. From A Child Is Born *(Dell Publishing Company, 1990), used by permission.*

of conception, gestation, and birth, but, by implication, their essential or self-evident, if also somewhat opaque, meanings, as if the camera itself were simply a vehicle for the transmission of natural truths and Nilsson a privileged scribe.[2] And then there is the use to which these and other similar images have been put over the course of the past decade. Nilsson's "full color fetal portraits"[3] have been widely circulated by prolife activists as vivid visual evidence of what these activists regard as the biological facts of fetal life—facts that have been substantiated, or so they argue, by the science of fetology and that reveal beyond reasonable challenge the specifically and self-evidently human quality of that life, its autonomy and identity as an innocent, vulnerable, and unique preformed human being, a miniature version of you or me.[4] The fetus, when viewed, is now heard to speak a truth about itself—indeed, in this video is heard, literally, to speak its potential or speak as it might at age three or four or five through laughter. But no image is self-evidently what it is, no meaning a simple matter of natural fact brought to light, as in the case of the fetal form, by scientific advances in either fetology or fiber optics. If the fetal form speaks, it is because that form is itself a densely constructed figure of speech—a figure in and through which is condensed and articulated a full range of historically, culturally, and ideologically embedded values, assumptions, claims, and contests. As such, its meaning cannot be suspended by fiat nor easily reinflected. Although the concluding segment of the video may attempt to construct the imaginary both within and against the rhetoric of the fetal image to tell a story of refusal and regret, in the end that story gives way to another, more potent, public tale of self-mutilation and murder.

In the video's last segment, then, a child's laughter, along with the image of an eighteen-week-old fetus raising its hand in an attempt to shield itself from our peering gaze, stages our entrance into a world of condensed and contorted meanings. The image of the fetus becomes the image of a woman, again behind glass, sucking water as does fetal life in utero, her features wet and distorted. Banter begins of the sort one might hear between a mother and child—and yet the affectionate playfulness we generally associate with such banter assumes rather sadistic overtones after what we believe we have just witnessed: "I hear you," a woman's voice taunts, "I see you. Bye-Bye, Baby." This time, the image of a seven-week-old fetus, fifteen times its actual size, fills the screen before us, its hand moving as if to wave. "Child of my imagination," the narrative continues, "you will never be child. Flesh of my flesh, you will never be flesh." The image of the seven-week-old fetus is transformed into its eighteen-week-old counterpart, which in turn becomes the woman behind glass. We are dispatched to the moment of conception as sperm cluster about an ovum, spectators to creation and the creation story contained within it—the division of the original flesh and its subsequent corruption through an assertion of will. "Dismember. Disintegrate. Dissolve," a voice instructs, and thus is marked our fall both figuratively and literally.

With this imperative, we are forced downward through the passage that was our entry into the exotic interiors of biospace, expelled from the body even as we become spectators to an expulsion, a live birth that is nevertheless not one. Labored breathing attends our passage. "These are dangerous times," we are told, and although we might wonder precisely for whom they are dangerous, the visual text leaves little room for question. A fetus/baby emerges into surgically gloved hands, hands that will also appear in the next several frames to reverse their action and assist as the body draws this disappearing life back into itself: "a memory of flesh." We see a woman lying on her back, writhing in pain and, finally, rock salt floating once again upward through water into a hand positioned at the top of the screen. With the iteration of a feminist politics now rendered parody, our excursion of discovery ends: "My body . . . my choice . . . my childlessness."

III

What makes this video make the sense it makes? What social, histori-cal, cultural, and ideological spaces does it inhabit and produce? The program notes that accompanied at least one screening of *S'Aline's Solution* describe it as "affirm[ing] a prochoice stance while acknowl-edging the loss incurred in an aborted pregnancy."[5] Audiences of mixed race and gender have nevertheless found the piece both disturb-ing and confusing, and have tended, in postscreening discussions, to divide, more or less generationally, according to one of two readings in their accounts as to why. Slightly older viewers, for example, have not tended to recognize the stance the video adopts as "prochoice" in any substantive or meaningful sense, and point to the dissonance that is produced by the spoken, visual, and audio texts. The rhetoric of the images and the sense of suspense and impending doom invoked by the sound track together collide with and ultimately subvert the ostensibly prochoice rhetoric that initiates and closes the action. In addition, there is the "discourse of loss" that the piece articulates in and through the fetal form. Within the current culture of abortion, "loss" or its ab-sence has been deployed to reframe the meaning of the practice and, in effect, functions as an argument against abortion even when invoked within a prochoice context. Recall for the moment the discussion in chapter 2 regarding the "emergence" in the early 1980s of "post-abortion stress syndrome." This condition was said to afflict women after they have had abortions, in some cases years later, and included among its vast range of indications guilt, remorse, despair, with-drawal, a sense of helplessness, a preoccupation with babies, self-destructive behavior, diminished powers of reason, diminished work capacity, anger, rage, hostility, and child abuse. Although this "con-dition" eluded the classificatory efforts of public and private health officials, it nevertheless captured and, for that matter, continues to capture the public imagination because it allays popular fears and anxieties with respect to what have been dramatic shifts in the organization of sexuality, parenthood, reproduction, and the family over the past two decades. Women may act in willful defiance against their essential nature as women, the syndrome seems to suggest, but nature nevertheless persists. On the other hand, women who experience no sense of loss or remorse following aborted pregnancies, initially construed within popular discourse and debate as callous, hard, selfish, capricious, or "unwomanly," were instead depicted by the late 1980s as maternally illiterate or simply ignorant about the true nature of fetal life. This could be corrected, it was argued, through ultrasound imaging, the assumption being that after having viewed the fetus she was carrying, a woman would realize its essential or true nature as a preborn child, bond with it, and forgo abortion.[6]

Despite authorial claims to the contrary, therefore, somewhat older viewers have tended to read *S'Aline's Solution* as a prolife text. In contrast to this reading, younger, college-age viewers—viewers who came of age in Reagan's America or during a period that saw the culture of abortion profoundly transformed—have tended to find the video's multitextual renderings of both the meaning and implications of abortion unproblematic and unproblematically prochoice. What these viewers have found troubling is the practice itself, *given* its apparently obvious meaning and implications. Although necessary, abortion is as the video, in their reading, accurately depicts it—violent and dangerous, the disruption of "natural" biological processes that naturally disturbs psychological ones and produces confusion, remorse, guilt, and despair. Curiously, however, such suffering has been construed by these viewers not only or primarily as punishment, as the price women must pay, or a "residual motherliness" persisting in the absence of something to be mothered. That women might suffer the decision to terminate a pregnancy both before and after making it is read as evidence of a certain moral sensibility. Within the context of a discourse that, at least in principle, has no way of registering moral seriousness or generating moral argument—and such is the case with liberal discourse about abortion—psychological hesitation and uncertainty have come to function as their sign and substitute. Both were marshaled to counter charges heard frequently throughout the 1980s that women have abortions for reasons of convenience, and are precisely what now "legitimates" choice in public discourse and debate. It is, then, primarily through the transposition of guilt and choice that those in this second, younger group of viewers apparently "resolve" what their somewhat older counterparts regard as the contradiction between the prochoice rhetoric that frames the video's visual text and the rhetoric of the text itself. The question is whether, and in what sense, such a "resolution" works to recuperate rather than reinscribe the discursive terrain prolife representations, meanings, and practices have come to dominate. Or, to put this question more generally, is it possible to reinflect signs already in circulation, as one might argue this video attempts to do, for another political end? And, with particular respect to the video, to what extent can arresting images of the fetal form floating free in space, the trope of discovery, or a particular mode of visual argumentation, rooted in the authoritative power of science and medicine, be reappropriated given that they anchor and are anchored in and by another set of stories having to do with the perilous plight of the prenatal iterated throughout the past decade in the streets, courts, and clinics?

Although *S'Aline's Solution* does not claim to be a "medical document"—to represent the "medical reality" of abortion or the truth of natural facts, as does, for example, *The Silent Scream*—an aura of medical authority, generated primarily from the images, nevertheless suffuses the text and lends it credibility. Although we may query the video's politics or its broader political implications, we do not question where we have been or what we have seen, let alone how we have come to see it. We assume, and are encouraged in the assumption, that we have entered a female body and there witnessed a violent and traumatic interruption of natural processes. But suppose it were the case, as indeed it is, that the opening sequence of the video transports us into the biospace of the genitor rather than the genetrix, and that we travel, initially, not through or along the fallopian tubes, as we might have imagined, but up the male urethra. Suppose it were the case that the sequence of images we are inclined to read as a saline abortion turns out to be ejaculation, that the white fluid we construe as the saline solution is seminal fluid, that our expulsion from the body in the concluding frames of the video is not through a birth canal, but, again, through the urethra as ejaculate. Although the video maker does not acknowledge the use of footage from *Nova's Miracle of Life*, all of the images of the exotic inner space of the body, as I mentioned earlier, are drawn from this production.[7] And with the exception of those images of reproductive organs unmistakably female—a swollen follicle, a ripe ovum, the outermost fringes of the fallopian tubes—it is in and through the male body that this drama of fetal life and death unfolds.

So much for the given, the unquestionable, and the self-evident. What permits us to read ejaculation as a violent, traumatic, distinctly unnatural rupture of natural processes is not only our general illiteracy with respect to the interior functioning of bodies—this is to be expected—but our illiteracy coupled with powerful prior notions and anxieties themselves shaped by a larger public discourse and culture of abortion about what the practice is, means, and entails. Deeply embedded assumptions about who and what women are and are for; the increased public presence of the free-floating fetal form; the construction of fetal independence and dominance, both medically, in the context of advances in the "new" science of fetology, and legally, through the aggressive implementation of fetal protection statutes; new obstetric technologies such as ultrasound, along with increasingly routinized genetic screening and subsequent shifts in the management of pregnancy and birth; the development of new reproductive technologies and their attendant discourses of female desperateness and deviance; clinic bombings and numerous kidnappings and murders of physicians; the emergence of conditions such as postabortion stress syndrome; legislative and judicial struggles over abortion access; the perceived dissolution of the nuclear family; the antifeminist backlash; the production of *The Silent Scream* and such highly popular movies as *Look Who's Talking*, *Baby Boom*, *Three Men and a Baby*, *Aliens*, and *The Hand That Rocks the Cradle*—all of these things together constitute the contemporary grammar and culture of abortion, and over the course of the past fifteen years have together worked a powerful restructuring of how we experience, understand, configure, and speak the practice. *S'Aline's Solution* produces and is produced by this culture; indeed, it is this culture that allows us to connect the dots, to organize and assemble a collection of slogans and a collage of otherwise unidentifiable bodily processes in a way that creates a coherent and compelling, if also deeply disturbing, tale. It is, in the end, what enables us to tell the story we believe we are being told, what predisposes us to see in a moment of orgasmic pleasure a saline solution or final solution, genocide.

We could, of course, venture the telling of another story. Knowing now what the images in the video "really" are, knowing that ejaculation is being deployed as the visual representation of abortion, we could embark on another excursion of discovery and attempt to rescue the narrative, force from it a certain irony, submerged logic, or set of stories perhaps more complicated, subversive, and politically clever than the story we assumed we were being told. Drawing on "subcultural" figurations of abortion as well as Old Testament allusions that riddle the narrative, we might insist that the video invites us to read against the deep structure of contemporary formulations of the dispute. It renders the female body, as much popular discourse and debate regarding abortion renders it, utterly irrelevant. In so doing, however, the video makes conspicuous the absence of this body, the gestating body, in contemporary renderings as well as its construction as both an abstraction and aberration. Within public discourse, the body that signifies and is significant, that is generative and in its generation produces both meaning and value, is the (heterosexual) male body. According to biblical accounts, of course, it is the original flesh, the flesh from which all flesh originates and to which all flesh is subsequently subordinate. In the beginning there is but one flesh, and it is an act of will that divides it—Eve eats from the tree of the knowledge of good and evil and is subsequently expelled from the garden along with her mate and master, Adam. Through her transgression is initiated their fall from grace and subsequent expulsion; it marks the separation of heaven and earth, the alienation of body and soul, the opposition of a flesh once one.

With the opening of the video, we enter and occupy the body of the genitor, the original flesh, only to be expelled from that body at its end as the result of choice: "I choose, I chose, I have chosen." The choice that is abortion is an act of insurgence; it refuses the destiny of sperm and women's own destiny, which is derivative, which is dependent upon sperm for its fulfillment. It disrupts an original unity uncontaminated by sexual differentiation, disrupts the natural order of things, subverts signification, destabilizes meaning and value. It entails the dismemberment and disintegration of the generative body—indeed, mutilates the one body and produces two. In this version of the video, state-of-the-art imaging technology is deployed to tell a biblical story, the story of creation and the fall, but, shifting Testaments now, also a story of possible redemption, conventionally regarded within contemporary prolife religious discourse as embodied in the figure of the fetus. While signifying women's restless agitation against a preordained natural order, the aborted fetus is also a symbol of sacrifice for prolife activists, offered for the redemption of both Man and America.[8] Recognizing her

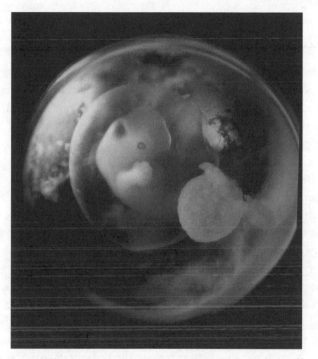

Copyright Lennart Nilsson. From A Child Is Born *(Dell Publishing Company, 1990), used by permission.*

relationship with the fetus she carries, (S')Aline's solution is nevertheless to refuse its terms and thus forfeit redemption: "My body, my choice, my childlessness." The sense of impending doom fostered by the auditory text both frames this refusal and tells us something about its consequences.

What is curious about this reading of the video is that while it remains true to the apparent truth of the images or departs from the point we assumed we were departing from originally, from the biologically given, it seems nevertheless to be more figurative, interpretive, or inferential than the drama the piece appears to present, the drama of fetal life and death. This is due, at least in part, to how conspicuous the play becomes with this alternative reading between what the images "are" and what they "mean." In order to make the visual text make sense, we are required to perform a series of translations, the obvious performance of which clearly circumscribes the persuasive force of the sense we make. Next to a story that seems simply to tell itself, to image the natural and through this imaging bring to light matters of fact, any account we might proffer, although plausible, will seem both contrived and interested, one story among many possible stories, but none of these is the "real" story in some objective or self-evident sense.

The point, of course, is that both stories—the tale of innocence imperiled and that of innocence lost—are densely constructed, and although the latter appears to be more obviously constructed than the former, quite the reverse is the case. Through its ostensible use of medical-scientific and visual technologies—or footage from the *Miracle of Life*—the video appears to present a biological rather than social text, the natural facts of (a saline) abortion, and acquires a certain symbolic power as a result. That we are reading the biological entirely through the lens of the social becomes obvious when we realize we have been trekking about the male reproductive tract, spectators to an event we do not typically think of as either violent or traumatic. But even were this not the case, even were we "actually" situated, as we are encouraged to assume we are, in a female body, and in the general proximity of a saline abortion, we would still be tracking and reading the social. Peering technologies such as ultrasound and fiber-optic imaging do not simply turn the inside out, render the oblique transparent, or extend our vision to reveal the elusive secrets of nature. Technologies themselves do not peer; they are *instruments and relations* that facilitate or obstruct but, above all, construct "peering," indeed, instruments and relations that do not simply uncover meaning, but inscribe and enforce it.[9] Likewise, "peering" is not itself a benign, impartial, disinterested, or disembodied activity, but is both mediated and situated within interpretive frameworks, points of view, and sets of purposes—how else is the body "revealed," read, or made legible to an observing eye? As I have suggested in chapter 1, what we see is inseparably linked to and utterly dependent upon how we see. And, in the case of this video, how we see is clearly constructed in and through the contemporary discourse and culture of abortion. The issue is not what these images are "really" images of. The issue is, rather, "how" these images mean what they mean, and how they have come to mean it.

IV

Although *S'Aline's Solution* claims to represent only one woman's struggle to come to terms with an aborted pregnancy, the terms in which that struggle is figured illustrate the degree to which popular discourse and debate over the course of the past decade have profoundly transformed the perceptions and practices that together constitute abortion. In the era immediately preceding *Roe v. Wade,* "criminal prosecution, morbidity, and maternal as opposed to fetal mortality" constituted the cultural anatomy of the practice or the terms in which it was conventionally known, understood, constructed, and experienced.[10] Women struggled for control over their reproductive lives, despite legal constraints and life-threatening conditions, and many women died—indeed, women in the United States died yearly from illegal abortions in greater numbers than did U.S. soldiers in Vietnam, and black women died at eleven times the rate of their white counterparts.[11] Throughout this era, abortion was also the privileged sign of another, always present and constitutive, but submerged, set of meanings having to do with women's sexual freedom, autonomy, and agency; notwithstanding contemporary distillations, "My body, my choice" has never been only or simply a question of protecting or expanding the procreative options of the naturally reproducing white heterosexual body. In *Roe v. Wade,* the Supreme Court chose, predictably, to circumvent the potentially more radical meanings of legalization by situating the practice within a medically defined and controlled framework. Similarly, reform groups and family planning organizations worked methodically to both contain and conceal them.[12] Clearly, however, the radical challenges potentially posed by legalized abortion to traditional gender identities and sexual relations were hardly lost on neoconservatives and their New Right and fundamentalist affiliates, and, over the course of the past decade, have inflamed popular debate while themselves being recast and transformed in the process.

Thus, for example, in the presence of the fetal form and the theater of charges animating it of murder and selfishness as well as neglect and abuse, the expanded sense of freedom and power that abortion has afforded many women in allowing them to take hold of their lives is only rarely mentioned, and then often in a passing whisper. In the public vernacular of abortion, freedom and power have an at best pejorative resonance and function, when invoked, as a potential indictment of all women in the phantasmatic rendering of one—the casual, capricious, career-minded woman who has abandoned hearth and home and kills without conscience. Even those who champion choice have shifted registers and now speak not of freedom or power, but of dire choice and desperation. Abortion is cast as a grim and grievous practice, and the woman who has one as either psychologically troubled and morally ambivalent or irresponsible and promiscuous—in either case, as a victim of a regrettable if at times unvoidable violence. Finally, within this register, "choice" too has been transfigured as the maternal body, driven by the needs and interests of others, has increasingly displaced the self-regarding sexual one as its referent. A poster at the 1989 march on Washington for abortion rights graphically depicts this shift: pictured under the boldly lettered caption "Pro-choice not Pro-abortion" and set against a black background are the lower abdomen and spread legs of a woman giving birth. An attending physician, midwife, or friend is grasping the partially emerged infant under its arms, both easing and enabling its final moments of passage. The title of the portrait is in script; it reads, "The Miracle of Birth."

Although this portrait attempts, like *S'Aline's Solution,* to recuperate terrain now dominated by prolife meanings and representations by articulating what has come to be regarded as a more complex or morally textured stance with respect to "choice," in the end it reflects only their ubiquity and strength. Indeed, in the end, both video and portrait succeed only in reinscribing and fortifying these meanings—in the case of the latter, by situating the woman who is giving birth, literally, outside the frame. We see a fragment of her body, her pelvis, and only as the stage upon which a separate and determining life is enacted. She is not liberalism's bounded individual, the one who is indivisible, who cannot be divided and, thus, the one who is able to act or exercise choice; rather, she is represented in this portrait as divided and dividing, the one who is acted upon and through.[13] Similarly, in the video, although woman and fetus are both within the visual frame, they do not share the same frame, the same body, or the same story. The fetus floats free, a discrete and separate entity, outside of, unconnected to, and, by virtue of its ostensible or visual independence, in an adversarial relationship with the body and life upon which it is nevertheless inextricably dependent. It tells its own story, is an effect of power or a figure of speech that has been both authored and authorized in the courts, clinics, and culture at large and that cannot be silenced or appropriated in the same way that women's stories and struggles are in its presence. In its presence or a context in which the image—fetus—is (mis)read and thereby constituted as the thing it signifies[14]—baby—women's stories and struggles can be heard only as thin rationalizations, "excuses," digressions, or, in the case of the video, deranged utterances of a disturbed nature.

In the end, the very terms in which this video attempts to tell its story of loss work both to indict and to silence it, for notwithstanding their general acceptance within the present culture of abortion as more scientifically informed and morally complex,[15] these terms are, nevertheless, reductive and simplifying and reflect the extent to which prolife meanings, categories, and representations have so saturated public discourse as to now seem part of the fabric of fact. For a genuinely informed and complex story of abortion to be heard, the speech that would render women speechless must be interrupted. This entails, among other things but most basically, interrupting "the visual discourse of fetal autonomy"[16]—developing a vocabulary of relationship that reembodies the disembodied fetal form or resituates the gestating fetus in a uterus, the uterus in a body, and the body in social relations, thereby re-membering what is otherwise dismembered and, in every respect, truly in a perilous state. Pregnancies, when they occur, occur in women's bodies. For those who champion "choice" to lose sight of this simple and obvious, yet profoundly radical and consequential fact in a post-1980s struggle for reproductive freedom would be finally to surrender the possibility of freedom. If these are dangerous times, as the narrative of the video at one point asserts—and they are—*S'Aline's Solution* could itself be read in the end as a striking if sobering illustration of why.

4 / Reproducing Public Meanings:
In the Matter of Baby M

I

By the time Judge Harvey Sorkow handed down his ruling upholding the surrogate agreement in the so-called Baby M case, much of the drama that had suffused the seven-week trial had been spent. For weeks, major newspapers had featured pictures of Baby Stern/Whitehead being passed from birth mother to biological father with state troopers at hand to ensure an orderly transfer. Often accompanying these pictures were character sketches and lengthy life histories of the principal players in the dispute. The viewing public had been invited "to contemplate with anguish the constant pressures and conflicts [the baby would] confront throughout her growing years"[1] and to consider which of the two families seemed best able to provide for this child, who, experts claimed, would eventually suffer some kind of psychological trauma no matter how the dispute was resolved. Was it in the best interest of Baby M to be placed with a family of stable, mutually supportive, educationally motivated professionals, living "private, quiet, unremarkable lives," or could the full range of her anticipated needs be met by high school dropouts, one a sanitation engineer, alcoholic, and subordinate male, and the other a former stripper with dyed hair and suicidal tendencies?

By the time Judge Sorkow issued his landmark decision giving sole custody of the child to the unremarkable Sterns, the commercial practice of "surrogate motherhood" was under close and critical scrutiny in a variety of arenas. Hearings had been scheduled in state legislatures across the land to assess the status and commercial aspects of such agreements and to begin consideration of other, similarly "novel," forms of reproductive technology that, like surrogacy, existed in "legal limbo." Juvenile-rights attorneys had begun to assess the implications of "biomedical advances" for laws on adoption, child custody, and parental rights, and public policy analysts had begun calling for stricter guidelines and tighter regulation of what, upon closer inspection, looked like "bucks for babies" deals. Journalists had reviewed the "disturbing" challenges such advances posed for American society, while psychiatrists pondered, scholars wrestled, and women's rights activists marched—some specifically on behalf of Mary Beth Whitehead's natural, "maternal" claims, others to draw attention to the continued degradation and oppression of women reflected in the twisted character of the proceedings and the specious testimony of "expert" witnesses regarding Whitehead's alleged personality disorders.[2] The issues were many and confused, and conventional understandings and assumptions were destabilized. If the proliferation and deployment of new reproductive technologies had "brought society to the brink of something almost like the atomic bomb," as the former president of the British Medical Association, Sir John Peel, put it, Baby M seemed clearly to indicate the first sign of serious fallout.[3]

It had not been entirely unexpected. In a case that preceded the Baby M trial and concerned the brokering of surrogate agreements, the Kentucky Supreme Court had cautioned that surrogacy and other "novel" solutions to infertility offered by advances in biomedical science were ushering in a confusing "new era of genetics." Earlier in the decade, Doris J. Freed, head of the American Bar Association's Family Law Section, had likewise warned that the deployment of these new technologies would provoke a "moral, social and legal nightmare."[4] Judge Harvey Sorkow, then, seemed merely to be echoing these widely held sentiments when he observed in his ruling that reproductive science and technique, although presenting "awesome opportunities," were rapidly outpacing society's ability to cope with them in a coherent, effective fashion. Indeed, so technically exceptional was the phenomenon of "surrogate mothering," Judge Sorkow maintained, and so distinctive were the family forms beginning to emerge from it, that no existing law pertaining to adoption, custody, or the termination of parental rights could be considered applicable or relevant to resolving the dispute. What lay before the judge as he apparently saw it was unsettled legal frontier. Upon this frontier, his would be one of the first flags raised, and raise it he did in the name of the father: "But for him there would be no child," wrote Sorkow. "The biological father pays the surrogate for her willingness to be impregnated and carry *his* child to term. At birth, the father does not purchase the child. . . . He cannot purchase what is already his."[5]

Sorkow's efforts to settle the legal bush were more or less undone within a year when the New Jersey Supreme Court reversed many of his findings upon appeal. While acknowledging surrogacy's novelty as a reproductive arrangement, the court moved to resituate the practice within the framework of existing state law and public policy, arguing that its principal objective was "to achieve adoption through private placement." Read in the idiom of adoption, surrogate arrangements entailing payment appeared to the court to be a form of baby selling— "illegal, perhaps criminal, and potentially degrading to women."[6] Also recast with this shift was the surrogate contract or "prebirth agreement" delimiting the terms of collaboration between a "surrogate" and "commissioning couple" and providing specifically for the termination of a surrogate's parental rights and claims. Such agreements, the court maintained, were coercive and unenforceable. In private-placement adoption as well as adoption through an approved agency, "the formal agreement to surrender occurs only *after* birth . . . and then, by regulation, only after the birth mother has been counseled."[7] Invoking what it took to be settled interpretation of New Jersey law, the court contended that surrender of custody and consent to present one's issue for adoption were only rarely irrevocable; indeed, when rescinded early enough, such agreements were generally considered irrelevant. Finally, and in some respects most essentially, the court maintained that surrender of custody and consent to adoption were binding only when both were made "knowingly, voluntarily, and deliberately," or in a manner, it argued, that neither could be in the case of surrogacy, given the terms and circumstances likely to accompany any prebirth agreement.[8]

> Under the contract, the natural mother is irrevocably committed before she knows the strength of her bond with her child. She never makes a

totally voluntary, informed decision, for quite clearly any decision prior to the baby's birth is, in the most important sense uninformed, and any decision after that, compelled by a pre-existing contractual commitment, the threat of a lawsuit, and the inducement of a $10,000 payment, is less than totally voluntary.[9]

Whereas Judge Sorkow had sought to stabilize destabilized practices, relationships, and identities through an act of founding—offering, as we will see in more detail shortly, an account of origins resonant, ironically, of the story the ancient Greek playwright Aeschylus tells in the *Oresteia* of the "original" founding—the New Jersey Supreme Court looked instead to conventional legal categories, cultural values, and public standards. In contrast to Sorkow, who, in the court's words, "had assumed [he] was writing on a clean slate," the higher court seemed to assume that it could merely read from one already given and inscribed.[10] Indeed, as the higher court framed the matter, Baby M was an occasion not for the generation of "new" meanings, but for the restoration of previously determined ones—and yet, of course, such matters are hardly so simple. Just as there are no clean slates upon which a court might simply write—no empty cultural spaces, no unclaimed, uncontested, or uncontestable fields of meaning—there are no plain slates from which a court might simply read. To paraphrase James Boyd White, legal texts are never "merely" read, they are always read only in the context of their making.[11] To "read" such a text is simultaneously to make it and, through it, a world; to read is to (re)configure social reality and relations or, in the case of surrogacy and the higher court's ruling specifically, to suture precisely those categories, identities, and relations rent by the practice.

If we situate the two rulings in the Baby M case side by side, we can see some striking similarities in the world that they produce, even while the sets of stories the two rulings tell in the process of producing that world appear on the surface to be dramatically different. The world Judge Sorkow "founds" beyond the present boundaries of law—a world organized and naturalized in terms of male prerogative—is the world that the New Jersey Supreme Court, positioned within these boundaries, "recovers" in the name of natural motherhood and maternal yearning. Sorkow ruled in the name of the father and the supreme court on behalf of the mother, but natural motherhood, traditionally at least, has presupposed a world of male prerogative or one in which paternal rights, although not absolute, are certainly primary.

The higher court, then, did not so much turn back Sorkow's findings as reframe them—and the difference, or so I will argue, is significant. Indeed, what I want to insist is that both rulings are equally constitutive, both are sites for the production of cultural meaning, both (re)consolidate cultural meaning even as they also simultaneously produce it. When Sorkow declares himself to be on uncharted legal terrain, the constitutive quality of his ruling is somewhat more apparent than when the supreme court finds for the "natural mother" and roots this finding in settled interpretation of New Jersey law. In fact, it is precisely because Sorkow's ruling is so obviously constitutive of a world without women that it must be turned back, at least ostensibly.[12] Following Foucault's insight, power operates effectively only to the extent that it can hide its own operation, and this is what Sorkow fails to do in rendering Baby M a "technobaby" of purely paternal origins.[13] And yet, in finding on behalf of the "natural mother," the supreme court's ruling is no less constitutive than Sorkow's; through a series of rhetorical moves, it stabilizes the notion of motherhood as natural and the biological discourse that grounds it as well as male prerogative. The ruling also simultaneously (re)constructs this notion of motherhood or circumscribes and naturalizes the social practices and relations that constitute what is called "mother" even while it appears only to be recovering it—conventional understandings of what constitutes "motherhood" are, after all, precisely what new reproductive practices—and surrogacy specifically, partial as well as gestational—have denaturalized, demystified, and thus thoroughly destabilized. Recovering the "natural mother" entails, *inter alia*, recovering—reconstituting as natural precisely what these new practices have revealed to be historically contingent and conditioned by relations of power.

"In every opinion," writes James Boyd White, "a court not only resolves a particular dispute one way or another, it validates or authorizes one form of life . . . or another."[14] The reading that I proffer in this essay of the original ruling in the Baby M case as well as the subsequent ruling that overturned it shares in this sense that the making of law is also the making of life—that law is not a neutral, disinterested, or discrete area of activity set apart from social practices and relations, but a politics or site of struggle, the means by which "one form of life" is authorized and codified against other forms and through both constructed.[15] Each ruling in the case of Baby M marks a particularly revealing instance of authorization and construction. A close scrutiny of both cases allows us to see not only how law simultaneously repairs and mystifies the relations of power that constitute "mother," "father," and "family" in the wake of their rupture while at the same time constructing these contested relations. It also allows us to see the ways in which the move to contain the proliferation of interpretive possibility is most centrally about containing the political possibility such proliferation necessarily forces open.

II

When Mary Beth Whitehead enrolled as a potential surrogate at the Infertility Center of New York in 1982, she assumed at least initially that she would function only as a host for someone else's genetic material.[16] When Bill Stern contacted the center some two years later in pursuit of biological offspring, he too assumed that the reproductive collaboration he was about to engage in would entail intricate biomedical maneuverings rather than sophisticated legal ones.[17] Expectations were not met in either case. The procreative alternative that produced Baby M—"traditional surrogacy," as it is now called[18]—required no real medical expertise and nothing more sophisticated, remarkable, or technologically exceptional than masturbation and the use of a syringe. Whitehead contributed an egg to Bill Stern's reproductive effort and was artificially inseminated with his sperm—but only after she had signed a maternity contract that suspended her parental claims to any child that might be produced as a result of the insemination and that held that this suspension was in the child's best interest. The truly novel feature of this procreative collaboration had little to do with the much-valorized efforts of medical science to negotiate the "reproductive imperative." The procedure that produced Baby M was legal rather than medical; it was designed to remedy issues of legitimacy and infidelity or potential malfunctions in the social body rather than perceived malfunctions in the physical one.

This important and obvious point was, if not lost on New Jersey Superior Court Judge Harvey Sorkow, certainly buried by him in the opening pages of his decision. In these pages, Judge Sorkow inscribes as a matter of fact a set of popular fictions that were iterated throughout the 1980s regarding infertility and part of the decade's deeply conservative pronatalist and racist agenda with respect to reproduction. Insofar as the construction of facts and the construction of law are mutually constitutive enterprises,[19] the judge's preamble not only frames the case of Baby M but tells us something about the terms in which it will be settled. Thus, he begins, for reasons having largely to do with lifestyle—delayed childbearing, increased sexual activity, and the attendant spread of sexually transmitted diseases—"large segments of our potential childbearing population" are now unable to fulfill "their intense drive to procreate naturally."[20] Although "adoption is often considered, . . . woman's . . . free choice to prevent [pregnancy or terminate it]" has resulted in "a dearth of adoptable children."[21] This has forced ever-increasing numbers of individuals to seek the assistance of medical science, with its ever-expanding arsenal of new conceptive techniques. According to the judge, these new techniques—and he includes "surrogate mothering" among them—provide the infertile with what may be the only truly viable means now available for obtaining a family, even while this form of "family" may itself be distinctly new and undefined. As Sorkow presents it, the rapid advance of reproductive science and technique has given society opportunities that are both "awesome" and as yet only partially realized. Whether these opportunities will fully evolve ultimately depends, in his view, upon the judiciary's willingness to define and direct the world they force open.[22]

Judge Sorkow's preamble presents the phenomenon of infertility as a seamless and self-evident reality. However, when infertility is read against a somewhat different social text, the "constitutive" quality of this reality becomes clear. Consider the court's observation that infertility is affecting an ever broader segment of society and the claim that gives this observation prescriptive force, that procreation is a biological necessity—a "drive that exists within the soul of all men and women"—and that those unable to realize it are both dysfunctional and desperate. Presented in this way, "infertility" establishes the need for the new conceptive technologies and legitimates their use; indeed, their necessity and legitimacy are placed beyond question. But there are other angles from which to view the phenomenon, and seen from these angles, infertility assumes a very different profile. It is the case, for example, that the actual rate of infertility in the United States has remained relatively constant over the last two decades. What has changed, particularly in the last ten years, is the expansion of possibilities for treatment, and much about the sudden appearance of an epidemic of infertility seems clearly related to the aggressive marketing of these treatments—themselves still experimental and of disputed effectiveness.[23] It is also the case that the incidence of infertility is one and a half times higher among poorer, nonwhite populations than in middle-class white ones, or higher in precisely those "segments of our society" in whom medical science appears to have the least interest and who, in any event, have the least access to its assistance. Contrary to the court's inference, moreover, infertility is attributable not only or even primarily to delayed childbearing, but to a diverse combination of social and iatrogenic factors: environmental pollution, exposure to hazardous toxins in the workplace, and unsafe working conditions in addition to inadequate health care provisions and sterilization abuse.[24] Finally, the "dearth" of adoptable children, which the court links to widespread abortion and contraceptive use, exists only if one is concerned strictly with the availability of "healthy" white infants.

What these "details" allow us to see is the way in which "infertility" is itself a contestable composition of specific and even predictable interests. The judge proffers an account that establishes the need for the new conceptive technologies, including surrogacy—they are "medical treatments" for a "medical condition"—while also featuring the novelty of these technologies. Surrogacy is about new science; new science is about a new world—not yet Huxley's *Brave New World*, in the judge's view, but new forms of life, relationship, and identity, the meanings of which have yet to be determined.[25] In other words, through his account of infertility and the rapid advances of science to treat it, Judge Sorkow has positioned himself and the case before him at the border of existing law and a new frontier. Arguing that the former is inadequate to the task of settling the latter—that law cannot inhabit a world its makers could not imagine and for which it was not intended—the judge crosses this border, thereby placing himself beyond the bounds of charted legal terrain: "It is submitted that at the time that even the most current adoption laws were adopted, no thought or consideration was given to the law's effect or relevance to surrogacy. . . . To make a new concept fit into an old statute makes tortured law with equally tortured results."[26]

Thus, Judge Sorkow is Columbus at Guanahani, the Pilgrims at Plymouth, Perry at the Pole. He will bring definition and order to the frontier that is reproductive technology and, as it was with those before him, his first gesture is an act of extended nomination. He issues a deed of possession, he claims this new land in the name of the father. Listen again to the judge's declaration: "But for him there would be no child," he writes. "The biological father pays the surrogate for her willingness to be impregnated and carry his child to term. At birth, the father does not purchase the child. . . . He cannot purchase what is already his."[27] Arguing in effect that the technobaby that is Baby M is born of the father's blood and scientific ingenuity, and only incidentally of a surrogate's/mother's/woman's body, Judge Sorkow (re)-invents paternity. This should not especially surprise us given that paternity has, at least traditionally, been regarded as the cornerstone of culture; and culture, new forms of relationship and identity, is precisely what the judge understands himself to be founding in the wake of new reproductive innovations.[28] Still, the irony of this founding moment is considerable, particularly if we situate Judge Sorkow's declaration against the story that the ancient Greek playwright Aeschylus tells in the *Oresteia* of the "original" founding, the founding of the law court of the Areopagus and thus of a new civilized and civilizing community of men—the founding, indeed, of Western culture.

III

In the *Eumenides*, the third play of the trilogy that makes up the *Oresteia*, Aeschylus celebrates the creation of a new civic order and vividly stages as part of that creation a dream that, according to classicists Jean-Pierre Vernant and Pierre Videl-Naquet, never ceased to haunt the Greek imagination. This is the dream of a purely paternal heredity, of a world if not without women than one in which women are both controlled and contained.[29] The drama opens at the temple of Delphi, to which the chief protagonist of the play, Orestes, has fled in hopes of enlisting the help of the god Apollo. Orestes has slain his mother, Clytemnestra, to avenge the death of his father, King Agamemnon. Although Orestes has acted by divine decree, he is nevertheless pursued by the Furies or Eumenides, female goddesses of an older age who champion the claims of blood ties, in this case Clytemnestra's claims, and who demand retribution for the matricide that Orestes has committed. The Furies surround him at Delphi, but with the aid of both Apollo and Hermes, Orestes is able to steal away and journey to Athens, where he appeals to Athena for absolution. Arguing that the case is too difficult for a single person to judge, Athena establishes a court of law and seats jurors to hear the dispute. The Eumenides contend that Orestes must give back blood for the mother blood he has spilled. Orestes' defender, Apollo, dismisses their claims, arguing that the maternal blood bond is insignificant: "Since the active regenerating function is exclusively male . . . maternal blood can never run in the veins of the son."[30]

> The mother is no parent of that which is called her child, but only nurse of the new-planted seed that grows. The parent is he who mounts. A stranger she preserves a stranger's seed, if no god interfere.[31]

Having asserted the procreative primacy of the father, Apollo moves to establish the truth of his assertion by reminding his audience of Athena's parentage, the goddess who was born not of woman but out of the head of Zeus:

> I will show you proof of what I have explained. There can be a father without a mother. There she stands, the living witness, daughter of Olympian Zeus, she who was never fostered in the dark of the womb yet such a child as no goddess could bring to birth.[32]

Sperm was thought by the ancients to originate in the brain or head of men, and thus to be a substance of mind, pure logos or reason.[33] Generated solely of mind, Athena herself represents its uncorrupted embodiment—she personifies reason and stands, by her own account, "always for the male." When the jurors' votes tie, she casts her ballot in favor of Orestes, thereby absolving him of the matricide. She explains:

> There is no mother anywhere who gave me birth, and but for marriage, I am always for the male with all my heart, and strongly on my father's side. So, in a case where the wife has killed her husband, lord of the house, her death shall not mean most to me.[34]

In founding order on the new frontier that is reproductive science, Judge Sorkow simply restages the Apollonian fantasy of reproduction with Baby M herself the living witness that "there can be a father without a mother." The technobaby that is Baby M is born of surrogacy, or what the judge (mis)identified in the opening pages of his ruling as a new reproductive technique. She is the "brainchild" of late-twentieth-century ingenuity, the personification of reason, the embodiment of rational choice, all of which are commonly regarded as the hallmark of reproductive science. Like Athena, who was born of Zeus, Baby M springs from the head of the man-god scientist and thus is as well "a child as no [woman] could bring forth." The judge's findings suggest, indeed, that for all practical purposes no woman did bring this techno-baby forth—for at birth, the court contended, Baby M had neither mother nor family.[35]

The yearning that produced Baby M—according to Judge Sorkow, the procreative drive—was Bill Stern's, not Mary Beth Whitehead's; male procreative desire is, after all, precisely what traditional surrogacy is deployed to facilitate, even while it is presented in popular discourse as something women do for other women. "But for him there would be no child," which is to say, sperm and sperm alone is the active or creative force and as such ensures right of access and ultimately of ownership—women themselves cannot hire surrogates.[36] Although Whitehead may have been related genetically to Baby M, her relationship, as the judge construed it, was from the beginning provisional and revocable by virtue of the contract she had signed. By virtue of this contract, her relationship could be neither meaningful nor maternal in any traditionally rendered sense of the word, given that "mothers"—or rather, "fit" mothers—do not sell their children or sell their bodies for breeding purposes. Whitehead was a surrogate or instrument of science, "a stranger [who] preserve[d] a stranger's seed," a "viable vehicle" for the fulfillment of what Judge Sorkow argued in the end was Stern's constitutionally protected right to procreate.[37] Indeed, in the end, "[Whitehead's] rights could be terminated because, as she had never really been the baby's mother, they had never existed."[38] She was someone who had made a deal—and broken it.

Positioned on the new frontier of reproductive science and beyond the bounds of charted legal terrain, Judge Sorkow's task, as he understood it, was to found new forms of life, relationship, and identity. What the judge did at this moment of founding was suture precisely that form of life and precisely those relationships and identities rent by surrogacy's deconstruction of the biological discourses grounding and legitimating conventional understandings of motherhood and family. In response to the discursive and material disorder produced by the radical transformation of reproductive practices and processes, Judge Sorkow (re)invented paternity or paternal law; through the warm, sensitive, humane, and victimized figure of Bill Stern, he naturalized and sentimentalized what is a form of life or set of social relations and practices rather than simply or even primarily a physiological relationship. At this founding moment, Judge Sorkow also (re)composed a corresponding form of family, organized around male prerogative and presupposed by it. Out of a novel reproductive arrangement he constructed an utterly conventional one—a good "old-fashioned," two-parent, economically self-sufficient "American" family with Bill Stern, the kindly paternal provider, and Betsy Stern, the legally "naturalized" mother, a pediatrician who would curtail her career to meet the infant's special needs and whose earnings, according to the court, "w[ould] supplement the family economy."[39] The techno-Baby M would live a privileged life in a recently purchased suburban home. She would be "enroll[ed] in a nursery school at about the age 3 not for learning purposes but for socialization, [grow up with an] opportunity for music lessons and athletics . . . , attend college . . . , [receive] professional counseling as required" and live, along with her parents, "a quiet, private, unremarkable life."[40] Such was the "new" world Judge Sorkow founded on the frontier of reproductive science and technique—and the same world that the New Jersey Supreme Court reconsolidated and reinscribed while ostensibly reversing Sorkow's findings upon appeal.

IV

The Supreme Court of New Jersey invalidated the surrogacy contract between Bill Stern and Mary Beth Whitehead, arguing that when surrogacy for payment is situated within the framework of existing state law and public policy, the practice constitutes a form of baby selling. Stern had paid for a product rather than a process—he had "purchased a child, or at the very least, a mother's right to her child."[41] The record with respect to such transactions or the commodification of labor, love, and life—a record the court presented as historical and legal as well as moral—was, in its view, absolutely clear. Resolution of the matter did not require the generation of "new" meanings, only the clarification and extension of previously determined ones—and yet, as I suggested earlier, in "reading" the record, the court was also simultaneously engaged in producing it. Like Sorkow, the higher court moved to restabilize the social relations and practices surrogacy disturbs and to found order in the wake of its disruption. In a manner reminiscent also of Sorkow, it did both through the telling of an ideologically familiar but no less constitutive tale of origins—a tale that sutures the biological and social or finds in natural bonds the basis for social ones. "In a civilized society," the court began,

> there are some things . . . that money cannot buy . . . In America, we decided long ago that merely because conduct purchased by money was "voluntary" did not mean that it was good or beyond regulation and prohibition . . . Employers can no longer buy labor at the lowest price they can bargain for, even though that labor is "voluntary" . . . , or buy women's labor for less money than is paid to men for the same job . . . , or purchase the agreement of children to perform oppressive labor . . . , or purchase the agreement of workers to subject themselves to unsafe or unhealthful working conditions. . . . There are, in short, values that society deems more important than granting to wealth whatever it can buy, be it labor, love, or life.[42]

This passage provides a rich account of ongoing social and political struggle reconfigured, however, by the court as "history" and condensed into a tale of collective moral restraint and mastery over the drives and desires of capital. In a "civilized" society, or what is called "America," meaning and value are stable; they are also stabilizing forces governing capital and restraining it from whence it would otherwise boldly go: babies are not commodities for sale nor women merely sites for their production, as commercial surrogacy would render each. But also contained in this passage is another kind of origins story, submerged but related to the dominant tale the court tells, having to do with natural motherhood and maternal yearning. For in the works of classical liberal theorists and critics alike, what tames and contains capital and makes possible a civil and civilizing community is the bond between mother and child.[43] This bond has traditionally been regarded as the original site of community—the prepolitical basis of collective life as well as the natural or constitutive basis for all social and moral relations. Characterized by the New Jersey Supreme Court in a subsequent section of its ruling as a force whose strength is second only to that of survival, it is, in the end, what permits us to become persons capable of treating other persons as ends rather than instruments.

In its ode to the birth of a civilized nation, the supreme court (re)establishes social order not only by (re)grounding that order in nature or the maternal bond, but by reinscribing, through that grounding, a thoroughly gendered division between public and private spheres, activities, and identities. Indeed, what the court founds is a world that is organized around and sustains male prerogative and paternal right—a world in which there is a public sphere of contract and market relations, of labor, exchange, calculation, distribution, and exploitation, conventionally defined as the world of equal and autonomous men, and a so-called private sphere of the family.[44] Traditionally regarded as the natural foundation of social life, the private sphere is, of course, where women, as guardians of order and morality, have been situated in the service of things concrete, particular, and bodily, as well as the family's male head. It is where women have engaged in their "distinctive" and "legitimate" life-giving and -preserving work, the unpaid work of childbearing and child rearing they are said to be fitted by nature to perform and whose performance has traditionally rendered them economically disadvantaged and dependent, subordinate, and, at least within classical liberal discourse, unfit for public life.

The court's founding tale recovers both the maternal bond or a conception of motherhood as something instinctual, natural, and ahistorical as well as the world this bond presupposes and produces, "an institutional arrangement that is widely held to be one, if not the, linchpin of women's subordination."[45] It also reinvents the conception it recovers insofar as the process of recovery is simultaneously and necessarily one of construction. In recuperating "natural motherhood," the court rebiologizes motherhood or naturalizes what surrogacy in particular and new reproductive practices more generally reveal as a thoroughly social and historically specific set of relations, constructed and conditioned by power. It (re)assembles and thus stabilizes conventional meanings of "motherhood" that surrogate practices disassemble by forcing deliberation with respect to whether the "real" mother is the contractual mother, the genetic mother, or the gestational mother. As Teresa de Lauretis argues with respect to gender—its construction "goes on as busily today as it did in earlier times"—so too obviously with "motherhood."[46] In recuperating "natural motherhood," the court authorizes and codifies as well as constructs against other possible meanings, practices, or formations who and what will count as "mother": Elizabeth Stern is the naturalized mother, but Mary Beth Whitehead is the "real" or "authentic" one.

Having recovered "natural motherhood" in the process of determining the status of commercial surrogacy, the court moved next in its judgment to instantiate it in the figure of Mary Beth Whitehead. Arguing that she had been harshly appraised by Sorkow as well as by some of the experts called upon to evaluate her mental and emotional stability, the higher court ruled that Whitehead's claims to the child she had borne—her genetic and gestational contribution—were equal in every respect to Stern's as the natural father. Although she had lied on numerous occasions and broken the law on numerous counts, breached a contract, and reneged on "a very important promise," she had acted, in the court's estimation, as any "natural" mother would have acted if forced to surrender her newborn.

> We think it is expecting something well beyond normal human capabilities to suggest that this mother should have parted with her newly born infant without a struggle. Other than survival, what stronger force is there? We do not know of, and cannot conceive of, any other case where a perfectly fit mother was expected to surrender her newly born infant, perhaps forever, and was then told she was a bad mother because she did not.[47]

Determining that Baby M's "parents were, and were to remain, her two biological parents,"[48] the court reconfigured the dispute between Stern and Whitehead as one regarding custody. It settled that dispute by awarding primary custody of the child to Stern. Although Whitehead was the "real" mother, Stern was the "real" and preferred parent. This judgment was perfectly consistent with the logic of the ruling's subtext regarding natural motherhood, and so too was its basis. Although willing to grant her visitation rights, the court refused Whitehead's bid for custody, citing precisely the same "evidence" or "expert opinion" that Sorkow had deployed in the process of erasing maternity and the higher court had rejected as harsh when restoring it. Sorkow had characterized Whitehead as manipulative, impulsive, irrational, irresponsible, narcissistic, domineering, and uneducated, and concluded that such a woman "could not be an impressive mother in general, or in particular, a good mother to Baby M."[49] Although the higher court argued that Whitehead had been if not a "good" mother, certainly a fit one—she had yearned for her newly born infant and struggled when forced to part with her—they nevertheless joined Sorkow in the conclusion that her personality would impede the child's growth.

> While love and affection there would be, Baby M's life with the Whiteheads promise[s] to be too closely controlled by Mrs. Whitehead. The prospects for wholesome, independent psychological growth and devel-

opment w[ill] be at serious risk. . . . [T]he evidence and expert opinion based on it reveal personality characteristics that might threaten the child's best development.[50]

In the view of the court, the kind of life that would best meet the full range of Baby M's many and special needs would be provided by her "natural" father and his wife, or, as they were described by the court, the loving, giving, nurturing, rational, open-minded, and financially secure Sterns. It was the Sterns who appeared to the court to approximate most closely what is called "family" and the Sterns who were once again constituted as such.[51]

V

Both rulings in the case of Baby M represent moments of instability and invention in the production of cultural meaning. Indeed, as we have seen, both rulings create and contain the social relations and practices that constitute what are called mother, father, and family in the wake of their rupture. Both contest for a world forced open, discursively as well as politically, by the radical transformation of reproductive practices and processes. Finally, both rulings stage the possibility—even as they also seek to foreclose it—of naming and figuring new forms of life, relationship, and identity. If the Superior and Supreme Courts of New Jersey produce the seemingly always already made—and much of this chapter has been devoted to mapping the process of this production—then clearly what is made can and must be made differently. As Jana Sawicki observes, "Although the new reproductive technologies . . . threaten to reproduce and enhance existing power relations, they also introduce new possibilities for disruption and resistance";[52] they represent new forms and practices of life that weaken the alibi of other forms and practices and place their terms at issue.

To exploit these possibilities positively, we must proceed on several fronts, mapping the unarticulated theoretical underpinnings and shifting complexities of contemporary reproductive contests and controversies. We must also generate concrete strategies of address that work to both cultivate and expand the shifting field of political openings that produce and are produced by these contests. As the new and, in the case of surrogacy, ostensibly new reproductive technologies are further developed and deployed, an already high-stakes struggle between op-

posing social forces over the reorganization of the processes and practices of contemporary life will only intensify. There are no guarantees
that efforts to interrupt or transform this reorganization will not be
cannibalized by the dominant structures that shape them—no guarantees and no definitive programs or settlements that might function as
such. Nevertheless, these efforts mark the nascent figurings of alternative worlds—a possible elsewhere—that are contained within but are
counter to the world currently being (re)produced in and through rulings like the ones handed down in the case of Baby M.

5 / Breached Birth:
Anna Johnson and the Reproduction
of Raced Bodies

I

On September 19, 1990, Anna Johnson, a black single parent of one, gave birth to a six-pound, ten-ounce, white baby boy in Santa Ana, California. Two days later, she surrendered custody of the boy to his genetic parents, Mark and Crispina Calvert, in order to avoid his temporary placement in a foster home while Orange County Superior Court Judge Richard N. Parslow Jr. reviewed Johnson's suit for parental rights and custody. The Calverts had contracted with Johnson the previous year to bring to term their in vitro fertilized embryo. In exchange for ten thousand dollars, Johnson agreed to be surgically impregnated with the Calvert zygote and to deliver the infant with whom she shared no genetic link once she was herself delivered. Claiming, however, that she had bonded with the fetus in the latter months of pregnancy and that the Calverts had, in any event, breached their contract both by defaulting on a prearranged payment schedule and by not caring adequately for her or the fetus—actions that, Johnson's lawyers maintained, constituted "fetal neglect"—Johnson sued for custody. "The child is not genetically mine, but I have more feelings for him than his natural parents do," she charged in a *Los Angeles Times* interview several months before the October delivery date. "If they are distant and uncaring now, what are they going to be like when he comes?"[1]

Maintaining that they had done even more for Johnson than they had been required to do by contract—they had "dr[iven] her to her doctor's appointments, g[iven] her money, brought her food, and asked how she was doing"—the Calverts contended that if anyone had been victimized financially or emotionally by this alternative reproductive arrangement it was they, not Johnson.[2] By their account, Johnson had acted in an increasingly unpredictable and exploitative manner: she demanded, for example, that they accelerate their payments on the ten thousand dollars owed her, which they did, and then threatened to keep the baby if they failed to produce the remaining balance. In their view, it was individual greed rather than maternal need that had motivated Johnson to sue for custody.

Circumstantially damning in this regard was not only the frequency with which Johnson had begun to appear on the popular talk-show circuit, but the public revelation, shortly after she filed suit, that she was facing two felony counts for welfare fraud.[3] Having allegedly failed to report her income fully for a ten-month period in 1989, Johnson was said to have received excess food stamps and AFDC benefits amounting to approximately five thousand dollars in overpayment. Although this was certainly not "the crime of the century," as Johnson's lawyer pejoratively characterized the district attorney's earnest prosecution of the case,[4] during the Reagan/Bush years welfare fraud had come to exercise a decidedly devestating hold on the national imagination and was both represented and regarded as the crime of the decade. Indeed, within Reagan's America, the always black, always urban, supposedly lazy welfare-dependent single mother or "welfare queen" functioned as a condensed symbol, deployed to "explain" not only the deeper pathology in black family life, but the destruction of the American way of life.[5]

Although the felony charges against Johnson clearly worked to discredit her testimony—lawyers for the Calverts lost little time in pointing out the wide shadow of doubt these charges cast on her integrity and the authenticity of her claims—in the end, I want to argue, it was largely irrelevant whether and in what sense they were actually true. Occupying and occupied by the category "black woman," Johnson entered the public discourse an already densely scripted figure whose deviance, whatever its particular form, was etched in flesh. Situated within a racially stratified society in which color is always already constituted and read through a received, if ever shifting, stockpile of commonplace images, Johnson entered the public discourse in terms whose meanings were narrowly circumscribed historically, symbolically, and politically, terms that rendered the integrity and authenticity of her speech already suspect.

In this respect, "her" story preceded and prefigured her. Set in postindustrial urban black America, reinforced by the visual terrain of popular culture and the discursive terrains of law and medicine, and iterated throughout the 1980s in the register of epidemic, this story had to do with the defrauding of social service agencies; with the long-term social and financial costs of "mentally and emotionally deficient" children perinatally exposed to crack cocaine; with the undoing of black masculinity and, as the media derisively depicted it, the "impending extinction" of the African American male;[6] with teenage promiscuity, pregnancy, illegitimacy, and the reproduction of a state-dependent and delinquent underclass; with child abuse and neglect, the erosion of family life, family values, and what the *New York Times* referred to as "one of the strongest forces in nature," the maternal instinct, through drug addiction, welfare addiction, and crime.[7] This story bore little relationship to the story Johnson herself would attempt to tell the court and was clearly irrelevant to her bid for custody. It was also and obviously partial: notwithstanding popular portrayals to the contrary, the majority of drug addicts in the United States are not black, but white and middle-class, and the rise in "illegitimate" births, said to have reached epidemic proportions during the decade among black women and teenagers, was rather among white women and teens.[8] Nevertheless, as part of the "cathected set of narratives signaled by the category 'black woman,'"[9] the tale of urban disorder and social decay would combine with an appeal to things genetic and natural to dominate the custody hearings. Not explicitly articulated, but both present and pervasive, it would be utilized not only to image the difference between truth and appearance, but to render Johnson's attachment to the white baby she had borne implausible and, thus, coldly calculating and confused.

II

As in the case of Baby M, the challenge for the Orange County Superior Court when custody hearings over Baby Boy Johnson were convened on October 9, 1990, was to restabilize conventional under-

standings of motherhood and family and thereby recontain the proliferation of meanings, identities, and relationships generated by the
panoply of new reproductive practices and, in particular, the practice
of gestational surrogacy. This the court would do in the process of
making a twofold determination—determining, on one hand, whether
gestational surrogacy was a form of baby selling (and therefore illegal)
and determining, on the other, whether and to what extent a gestational surrogate had claims over a child to whom she had given birth
but to whom she bore no genetic connection. In either case, the pivotal
question was the same: Was the genetic difference a difference that
made a difference?

Anna Johnson maintained that it did not. As one of her attorneys
plainly put the matter in court, "Genetics means crap in determining
parental rights," and his claim was not without considerable grounding in legal, medical, and popular practice. For example, while fashioned in a pretechnobaby age and concerned primarily with paternity
and adoption, California's 1975 National Uniform Parenting Act pre-
sumptively regards the "birth mother" as the "natural mother."[10] The
policy statement on surrogacy issued by the American College of Obstetricians and Gynecologists similarly endorses treating the birth tie
as the natural tie.[11] And then there is the reproductive discourse of the
decade—a largely reactionary, biologically reductive, and often contradictory set of narratives—elaborated in the distinct but clearly related arenas of abortion and infertility, shaped by the newly imaged,
newly "discovered" fetal "person" and directed toward refiguring maternal drives and desires, or what, in a postliberation era and through
the lens of this "discovery," appeared to have become recklessly and
grossly "disfigured."

Both abortion and infertility discourse constitute "maternal nature"
in and through gestation; indeed, gestation is regarded as precisely
what activates or brings fully into play women's essential maternal
core. This "core" or collection of drives and desires was represented
throughout the decade of the 1980s and within the context of both
discourses as being undeniably present in all women, even if it was
also dormant in some and disturbed, displaced, or frustrated in others.
Its assumed existence, as we have seen elsewhere in this book, not only
contributed to the construction of abortion as an especially heinous
crime against nature, an act of self-mutilation as well as murder, but
also lent legitimacy and urgency to the development of new techniques

and technologies for treating involuntary childlessness—a condition that would necessarily have to include *all* childlessness, whether chosen or not, as it certainly appeared to do by the decade's end.

Consider by way of example the report that appeared in the *New England Journal of Medicine*—the same week, ironically, that Judge Parslow handed down his decision in *Johnson v. Calvert*—announcing the development of innovative new techniques that would allow post-menopausal women to "reset their biological clocks" and "become mothers." The segment of the female population most fully and publicly featured as beneficiaries of these new techniques was not the 10 percent who had stopped ovulating in their thirties.[12] Rather, it was women who had "chosen" less traditional career paths and subsequently felt both loss and remorse—women, in other words, whose regret seemed to confirm, emotionally, what infertility spoken in the register of epidemic seemed to confirm biologically and scientifically: that however seductive professional life and ambition might initially appear, the ultimate end and reward of womanhood is motherhood. Here, as in much of the decade's discourse, anatomy and destiny were linked inextricably, even while the biologically uncompromising terms of that destiny could now be altered. That these women would be, as Anna Johnson was, genetic strangers to the embryos they would carry and the children they would later bear and rear hardly bore mention in the popular press; indeed, the question of genetic connection was virtually nonexistent as such.[13] The privileged story was the maternal story, gestationally rather than genetically spun and spoken.

If postmenopausal therapies in particular and infertility discourse more generally presuppose (and produce) a maternal nature that emerges in and through gestation, abortion discourse similarly assumes such a nature, although one that seems clearly to have gone awry given the prevalence of abortion: just as some animals kill their offspring when they are disturbed or in some way confused, so too were women killing theirs, "in restless agitation against a natural order."[14] A variety of explanations circulated throughout the decade as to the how and why of this disturbance, but shared among them was the sense, kindled by a 1983 study by noted bioethicist Joseph Fletcher and physician Mark Evans that appeared in the *New England Journal of Medicine,* that the problem lay in arousing repressed maternal drives or inciting recognition with respect to the true nature of fetal life and women's responsibility toward it.

In their study—itself based, as we saw in chapter 2, on only two un-related interviews—Fletcher and Evans argue that early ultrasound imaging of the fetal form can be used, in effect, as a remedial aid to stimulate maternal feelings in women who are equivocal about taking their pregnancies to term. According to Fletcher and Evans, viewing the fetus in utero appears to produce a "shock" of recognition in preg-nant women who have been unable or unwilling otherwise to perceive the fetus as a separate and vulnerable living entity that belongs to and is dependent upon them alone. This sense of recognition and, by impli-cation, responsibility, in their view, constitutes the stuff of maternal bonding, "the fundamental element in the later parent-child bond." Once this sense of recognition is aroused, they argue, women are more likely "to resolve 'ambivalent' pregnancies in favor of the fetus."[15]

Fletcher and Evans's speculations about the potential use of early ul-trasound testing to cultivate maternal nature and thus promote preg-nancy—their "visual bonding theory," as Rosalind Petchesky has referred to it—captured the imagination of prolife activists and com-munities alike: it inspired the production of *The Silent Scream* by the National Right-to-Life Committee,[16] intensified the mass circulation of fetal images in the latter years of the decade, and fostered legislative as well as judicial efforts to force pregnant women to view their fetuses prior to aborting them. Their speculations also prompted the practice among some obstetricians of incorporating ultrasound imaging at each monthly prenatal visit for the purpose of "helping [a] woman bond to her baby."[17] Finally, Fletcher and Evans's "visual bonding the-ory" could be deployed—although it was not—to account for the "shock" of recognition and growing emotional attachment Anna Johnson claimed to have experienced toward the fetus she was gestat-ing sometime after it quickened.

Recognizing that imaging practices produce the "fetus as baby" even as they appear only to reveal it as such, and keeping in mind as well the extraordinarily thin and narrow scope of Fletcher and Evans's "study," its pronatal agenda, and the larger political agenda it legiti-mated and was legitimated by, Anna Johnson could nevertheless be read through the lens of their study and the set of assumptions that ground it, indeed, the same lens and assumptions through which courts and legislatures throughout the land in the 1980s appeared both eager and poised to read millions of women, whether pregnant or only potentially so. She could be read as a woman initially "in denial," as a woman in whom maternal nature had been repressed, or as a woman whose initial sense of detachment from and ambivalence toward the fetus she was carrying was resolved "favorably" with the aid of monthly ultrasound testing, even though such testing was performed throughout her difficult pregnancy in order to track fetal growth rather than to facilitate "bonding."

The point here is that the way in which Anna Johnson was positoned and the terms in which she was read together reflect a subtle but significant shift in registers, a shift that can be seen and sharpened through a series of questions. In other words, if Johnson underwent precisely the kind of "conversion experience" during her pregnancy described and inscribed throughout the decade in dominant reproductive discourse as appropriately maternal and natural; if gestation aroused in her what postmenopausal therapies, among other reproductive interventions, assume to be and address as a deep, biologically rooted sense of maternal desire *regardless of genetic ties*; if her experience of herself, her pregnancy, and her relationship to the fetus she carried changed, as it typically does for women, once the fetus had quickened, what exactly did both the Superior and Supreme Courts of California, as well as the popular media, find so puzzling about her claim of having bonded with the child she produced and her bid for custody based on it? If "bonding" is regarded as something that happens universally and naturally; if the exception is considered that instance when a woman does not develop an attachment to the fetus she is carrying rather than when she does; indeed, if a woman's lack of maternal attachment is what is typically considered the stuff of scandal and deviance, what rendered Johnson's claim so remarkably queer, unfathomable, deviant, or unusual—in fact, so specious—as to inspire Superior Court Judge Richard Parslow to pathologize it as criminal, as a potential instrument for future emotional and financial extortion, and to dismiss it as groundless?[18]

Ostensibly, the issue from the court's point of view was Johnson's veracity—or, perhaps more accurately, her apparent lack of it. As Judge Parslow observed in his decision, "One of the problems with bonding is that it always involves credibility issues. If the only evidence is someone say[ing] 'I felt strongly towards the child, I bonded with the child,' you've got to take their word for it."[19] This the judge was clearly unwilling to do, noting that there was "substantial evidence in the record that [Johnson] never bonded with th[e child she gestated] until she filed her lawsuit, if then."[20] Giving birth was not in itself a constitutive sign of maternity. While acknowledging her gestational contribution—she provided "a place to carry the child" and was its "host"—the court went on to characterize Johnson's maternal attachment as provisional and, therefore, secondary. In Judge Parslow's words:

> Anna's relationship to the child is analogous to that of a foster parent, providing care, protection, and nurture during the period of time that the natural mother, Crispina Calvert, was unable to care for the child. . . . A foster parent provides care always understanding that the day may come when the mother of the child will once again be able to take the child and you have to give the child to the mother when she's met whatever conditions she has had to meet to have the child returned to her and walk away and live with it. That's the way it works. That's the way its worked for a long time.[21]

According to the judge, Johnson was neither conned nor coerced by the Calverts, but knowingly and willingly entered into a business agreement with them that circumscribed her relationship with the child she had consented to produce. This knowledge, he argued, the knowledge that "the baby would be exclusively the Calverts' when it was born," precluded the possibility of her having developed the deep, strong, meaningful, and abiding bond with it that she claimed to have developed. Invoking the testimony of Dr. Justin David Call, a child psychiatrist and pediatrician at the University of California, Irvine, and expert witness for the Calverts, Judge Parslow went on to distinguish Johnson's gestational attachment as primarily social rather than biological or natural. Bonds of the sort she insisted had formed, true maternal bonds, were likely to occur, he argued, only within the sanctity of a proper family unit, among "married mothers with husbands whose babies they carry."[22] Outside of this context, such bonding, in his view, was a matter of chance or choice:

> People that are married and get pregnant and plan for a child, that contributes to the mother's feelings toward the child she is carrying. And, in a situation, [Dr. Call] said, where the plan is from day one that the child is the genetic child of another couple but it's going to be given to that couple to raise exclusively when it's born means that there is less likelihood and should be less likelihood psychologically of a person carrying the child bonding with the child.[23]

Finally, the judge contended (again invoking Call's testimony) that, even in the unlikely event that Anna Johnson had, as she claimed, bonded with the fetus while gestating it, there was no clear indication, "no evidence whatsoever," that the fetus had bonded with her.[24]

As the court read the facts before it, who and what the fetus was and would become—its individual physiological and psychological identity—had more or less been settled genetically.[25] This, in its view, not only rendered the child the Calverts' product and property, but established between the child and the Calverts a bond that was both innate and indivisible—indeed, a bond that the court speculated would, were it severed, reduce the child, Christopher, to a state of genealogical confusion, imperil the development of his sense of selfhood, and eventually compel him later in life to seek out the deeper roots of his identity, his original family or place of natural origin. In the view of the court, the search for such origins or the desire to know the where, who, and how of our existence is itself a "built-in," natural, human instinct or drive, concretely expressed in the formation of families and, on a somewhat grander scale, the very science of genetics.[26] Insisting that a "three parent, two-mom claim was a situation ripe for crazy-making," Judge Parslow found that genetic connection alone both made and sustained a family unit and that gestation itself was merely an incidental in this case, a contractual moment in the constitution of that unit. Describing Mark and Crispina Calvert as a couple who had sought only to realize their most precious possession, their genetic heritage, a couple who between them could produce an embryo, but simply "ha[d] no place to carry it," the judge awarded exclusive custody of the boy to them, his genetic, biological, natural, and thus "real" parents, while relegating Anna Johnson to the status of surrogate carrier. That both of the "natural" parents had come by their "natural" parenthood in the most "unnatural" of fashions was apparently beside the point from the perspective of the bench. Speaking strictly in the register of the natural, the register that the court itself deployed, Anna Johnson's activities were considerably "more natural" than those the Calverts themselves performed. Nevertheless, in the interest of avoiding future psychological confusion and of consolidating this newly made yet "natural" family, further contact between Johnson and the child was terminated.

III

No one except Anna Johnson herself can say why she has waged this unseemly struggle.[27]

Judge Parslow asserted that of the many issues he was called upon to
disentangle in the case before him, race was not among them, and the
print media apparently agreed, noting that race itself had "played no
discernible role" in either the proceedings or the decision. Notwithstanding "the public prejudice," as William Steiner, court-appointed
guardian for the baby, reported it, "that Anna [was] a dumb welfare
mother trying to rip off the Calverts," in the estimation of the press,
the only moment of obvious racial impropriety during the hearings
was a remark made by Mark Calvert characterizing the custody battle
as "our blackest nightmare."[28] While recognized as tactless, this com-
ment was nevertheless excused as an indiscretion born of rage and
frustration. The Calverts, after all, were themselves an interracial,
hence self-evidently tolerant, couple—although not exactly brown,
Crispina Calvert, a Filipina, was not exactly white either. To the degree that anyone was identified as having a "problem" with race, that
person, ironically, was Johnson. As lawyers for the Calverts attempted
to present the matter, Johnson had been motivated to sue for custody
not, as she claimed, because of "maternal instincts" that had "just
come out naturally," but rather, they implied, because she fetishized
whiteness. "Have you ever told anyone that you always wanted to
have a white baby?" they inquired over the objections of her attorney.
"Considering that I'm half white myself," she replied, "no."[29]

Despite posttrial assessments to the contrary, the proceedings as
well as the decision in *Johnson v. Calvert* clearly worked to safeguard
the prerogatives of race and class privilege—indeed, both worked, as
Johnson's lawyer succinctly put it, to ensure that the white baby was
given to the white couple.[30] What invites and requires closer scrutiny is
how: What constellation of assumptions makes plausible the suggestion that the dark-skinned Johnson was simply lost in a dream of
whiteness—so lost in a struggle to achieve whiteness that she misled
and entrapped a couple whose infertility rendered them desperate and
vulnerable, indeed, so lost that she failed to see clearly who she was
and to whom the white baby she had "hosted" belonged even though
the answer had been scientifically established with DNA tests and was,

for many at least, visibly apparent? As Crispina Calvert asserted repeatedly in court and to the press, "He looks just like us."

Likewise, what narratives were at play and took flesh to facilitate the many curious inversions in this case? How did the judge, the Calverts, and the media, for example, escape what Johnson apparently could not, a preoccupation with race that courted pathology? What permitted the struggle she waged to be dismissed as "unseemly" when, typically, "foster mothers who grow attached to their charges and try to keep them are regarded with much popular sympathy and sometimes even succeed"?[31] And, speaking still of inversion, how did Johnson rather than the Calverts come to be positioned as exploitative and parasitic, when the Calverts paid Johnson what amounted to approximately $1.54 an hour—well below the minimum wage—to satisfy their genetic yearnings and gestate their zygote? Who exactly was the instrument of whom? Finally, what set of stories grounded the court's confidence, and apparently the public's as well, that they could read Johnson's "true" desires even if she herself denied or refused to speak them? What makes credible and coherent their conclusion that her custody challenge was duplicitous at best, evidence not of a change of heart or mind but of a failed moral character? And what evidence, other than her word, could Johnson have produced that would have qualified as such and substantiated her claim?

I suggested earlier that, as a black woman, Johnson entered the public discourse a densely scripted figure, positioned in and by a crude, if commonplace, set of racial caricatures and cultural narratives about "the way black women are." In the context of the court's allegedly neutral and neutralizing practice of "racial nonrecognition"—a practice that holds that "race" exists apart from the social and historical meanings that construct it, that assumes that one can acknowledge color without also reading it and that thus works to privilege precisely what it ostensibly prevents—both enjoyed unrestrained circulation, setting and circumscribing the terms in which her account could be rendered and heard.[32] Consider the felony charges of welfare fraud that were leveled in advance of the custody hearings and that haunted them throughout even though the infraction they alleged was shown later to have been the result of a bureaucratic mix-up of the sort for which state and federal agencies are legendary. These charges functioned to ignite, reinforce, and affix to the figure of Johnson "a constellation of ideas, images, and fears [already in circulation] about black women, the black family, economics, and cultural well-being."[33] They established as fact larger fictions of skin, or what Johnson's color already suggested could be assumed: *that she had been on welfare*, had, therefore, engaged in a form of "undeserved theft," and was, therefore, predisposed to ripping people off. The fact of welfare commingled with skin signified, among other things, moral depravity, lack of veracity, and capacity for deception.[34] It marked her as someone capable of deceiving the Calverts and exploiting their procreative yearnings in a coldly calculating fashion, for gain—indeed, as someone who lied rather than simply changed her mind.

If economic dependence, and the moral depravity it supposedly reflects, rendered Johnson's claim of having bonded with the white baby she had borne implausible, a related and equally powerful set of narratives having to do with the absent or arrested character of black maternal nature called into question her very ability to bond. Although these narratives have varied historically, they have figured black women's bodies and lives in one form or another since slavery, and share the assumption that black women are not only or simply maternally deficient: black women, while fertile, are rather "natally dead."[35]

The recitation of ostensibly high rates of illegitimate births, devastating images of babies perinatally exposed to crack or AIDS, equally arresting images of inner-city street slaughter, court-ordered implantation of the contraceptive Norplant to protect the current *and unconceived children* of women charged with "bad parenting"—these stories and others that circulated during the 1980s worked in conjunction with and as part of the dominant reproductive discourse of the decade to suggest that although black women can and do "breed" children, "they" neither possess nor display the instinctual drives necessary for mothering them.[36] As the court maintained with respect to Johnson— giving birth is not in itself proof of maternity—so too with respect to black women within the culture at large. In contrast to the maternally dormant and repressed white bodies depicted in abortion discourse or the maternally desperate and frustrated ones of infertility, the reproductive black body was figured within the decade's dominant discourse primarily in the coextensive if contradictory registers of absence and excess—as natally dead and thus dangerous, as boundlessly fertile and in need of containment. When black women fail so consistently to develop instinctual attachments to their own genetic offspring, the likelihood that one could or would develop bonds of the sort Johnson claimed to have formed with a genetically unrelated infant is remote. Indeed, it is, as the court's reading of Johnson through the medium and saturated meaning of skin clearly found it, unfathomable.

IV

Throughout this essay, I have been suggesting that the racialized meanings of skin set the terms in which the larger issues raised in the Anna Johnson case were addressed and settled. Color bears meaning and bears particular histories of meaning. Both enjoyed unrestrained circulation throughout the proceedings, indeed, both were clearly constitutive in shaping the particular way in which the court restabilized conventional understandings of parenthood and family disturbed by the practice of gestational surrogacy and the proliferation of relationships and identities accompanying it.

Having said this, I want also to suggest that the outcome of the case would not have been significantly different had Anna Johnson been white. Had Johnson been white, the central issues of race, class, and gender would clearly have been figured differently, and this difference might have recast the question of "extortion," for example, or resculpted the issue of veracity, or shifted the terms that informed the court's reasoning with respect to the child's "best interest." The outcome of the case, however, would have remained the same. The challenge before the court was to contain what signified as excess within the context of conventional understandings of parent and family or (re)naturalize and (re)authorize extant forms of life against other possible forms and formations. Containing excess or reauthoring and authorizing the familar is precisely what Judge Parslow's decision accomplished through the deployment of genetics, and it is also what his ruling would have sought to accomplish had the gestational surrogate been white. New reproductive practices and processes may force open the possibility of refiguring conventional cultural categories, identities, and relations: Judge Parslow "might have decided that while Johnson could not be considered a legal parent, she had a lesser right to share responsibility for and participate in the child's life."[37] But, as we have seen throughout this book, such practices and processes also work, not surprisingly, to foreclose this possibility, "to reproduce and enhance existing relations of power."[38] The court's findings in this case as well as the New Jersey court's findings in the case of Baby M worked to preserve the "natural" family (even as they also produced it) against "crazy-making" alternatives. And out of both conflicts the "natural" family emerged as a biologically rooted, racially closed, heterosexual, middle-class unit.

If the Baby M case intensifies our attention to how biological facts are deployed to facilitate the parasitical workings of class prerogative and male prerogative both shaped by particular imperatives about race in the construction of the "natural" family, the case of Anna J. allows us to track the parasitical workings and production of race shaped by class and gender. Although mapping the production and operation of class, race, and gender power in the context of rulings on such cases will not, in itself, interrupt this power, such a mapping can nevertheless serve the more modest but critical end of demystifying how such power works—and in that end lies a political beginning.

6 / "On Breeding Good Stock": Reflections on Herrnstein and Murray's *Bell Curve*

I

In September 1995, the *Los Angeles Times* carried a story whose headline read "San Diego Zoo Comes to the Aid of Embattled Iguana."[1] To a point, the story is a relatively familiar one. Inhabiting the shoreline of the U.S. naval base at Guantánamo Bay are giant rock iguanas. Of the many thousands of varieties of lizards that populate the world, the giant rock iguana has the distinction of now being among the most endangered and this, apparently, is where the San Diego Zoo comes in. The zoo's Center for the Reproduction of Endangered Species is conducting a multiyear, multimillion-dollar project funded by the National Science Foundation to study the iguanas of Guantánamo Bay. And as the *L.A. Times* reports it, the project has two goals: to rescue the iguanas from "the ravages of modernity" and to rehabilitate what researchers refer to as the iguana's "counterproductive mating habits."

Evidently, there is a tendency for dominant male iguanas to hoard females and viciously fight less assertive males for territory, with the result that the testosterone levels of subordinate males plummet: fewer males mate, fewer genes enter the pool, "modernity" continues its environmentally destructive march, and the iguanas become as the iguanas now are, endangered. To interrupt and, with time, remedy what would otherwise be the imminent extinction of the Guantánamo

Bay colony, the zoo's reproductive center has initiated a stopgap program that it calls "headstarting." As the *Times* article describes it, the zoo's "headstart" program entails removing "stud males" from the colony each year for a six-week period. This allows the testosterone levels of less assertive males to rise and fosters at least the possibility that they will then be able to engage in courting rituals and mate. The stopgap program also entails retrieving eggs from the Caribbean shoreline, hatching them at the zoo, conducting behavioral studies on the hatchlings, and then returning them to the bay after approximately eighteen months.

Forty-five hatchlings have already been "headstarted" at the zoo and, according to zoo officials, have thrived, growing twice as fast as their island-hatched counterparts. The question for researchers now is whether these initial and rapid "improvements" will be lasting or whether the acceleration of the "headstarted" iguanas will simply taper off and eventually "fade out" once they are returned to the colony and reassimilate. Finally, although "headstarting" has been both a modest and modestly successful intervention, the program still has its critics. According to the article, some researchers are concerned that the hatchlings will grow accustomed to their captivity and be unable to readjust to the wild, whereas others fear the hatchlings will grow overly dependent and attached to their keepers. To avoid both problems, the iguanas are apparently being fed a plant found at Guantánamo called "touch me not," and their contact with humans is "kept strictly to a minimum."[2]

Occupying the back pages of a Saturday-morning edition of the *Los Angeles Times* and told in a fashion that is jocular, in places, and obviously intended primarily to entertain, this story can nevertheless be read as offering a clear and chilling account of just how far the center of gravity has shifted culturally with respect to federally funded programs designed to redistribute access to societal wealth. The question seems glaring and unavoidable: What does it mean that what now circulates under the name "headstart" is a set of short-term strategies developed to remedy the reproductive dysfunctions of an endangered species in the Caribbean?

Of all the Great Society programs of the 1960s, Head Start is among the longest standing. It is also perhaps the most well-known and widely recognized program from this 1960s moment of racial redress. Head Start signifies in particular kinds of ways, in other words, and has a rich history of signification. This history of signification is not displaced, erased, or suspended with the zoo's appropriation and occupation of the practice called "headstart." It is rather refigured alongside and through it, which is precisely what makes the zoo's appropriation so deeply disturbing. The zoo's appropriation and occupation of the practice tells us something about contemporary contests over how entitlement programs and those whom these programs serve will signify and are currently signifying. Indeed, it suggests that "head start" now circulates as the sign for a set of temporary interventions designed in response to the "counterproductive mating habits" of *both* human and nonhuman populations. There is an easy slippage at play in this article between the human and the nonhuman. And when this slippage, this resignification, is situated in a larger social frame or in the context of the vitriolic debates that have gained force and breadth in the United States during the past decade over immigration, affirmative action, teen pregnancy, unwed motherhood, and welfare reform—indeed, over programs like Head Start—it is hardly entertaining. Such slippage is dangerous—even potentially deadly.

Contributing to the cultural shifts that have produced "head start" as a rescue operation for endangered lizards and also itself a clear reflection of these shifts is the late Richard Herrnstein and Charles Murray's highly controversial eight-hundred-page tome, *The Bell Curve*.[3] Published in 1994, *The Bell Curve* advances what Herrnstein and Murray contend are a truly revolutionary and scientifically verifiable set of claims that have, at least in their view, been politically censored to date.[4] Briefly, what they claim in this book is that each person is born with a fixed quantity of cognitive ability, the quotient of which constitutes his or her "IQ." What they claim to show is that there is an ascending slope of IQ scores in the United States that represents both a redistribution of intelligence and a growing class hierarchy. As Herrnstein and Murray read the figures, the United States is becoming increasingly more stratified, with groups dividing in terms of both wealth and intelligence.[5] "Success and failure in the American economy," they write, "and all that goes with it are increasingly a matter of the genes that people inherit." For this reason, predictably, "programs to expand opportunities for the disadvantaged are not going to make much difference."[6]

On the upper end of an emerging class divide is what Herrnstein and Murray refer to as the "cognitive elite," or individuals who share high

IQs, high incomes, and sound middle-class family values.[7] On the lower end dwells the "cognitive underclass," or individuals who are both "dull" and poor and disproportionately black; there are cognitively impaired white people, to be sure, but "the average white person," they contend, "tests higher than about 84% of the black population."[8] Although the authors find this stratification alarming, more alarming still are the fertility trends of each group. The cognitively gifted are reproducing at a torpid pace while the fertility rate of members of the cognitive, largely black underclass is steadily climbing and eclipsing that of their high-IQ, high-income, largely white counterparts. "We are ceasing as a nation to breed intelligence," wrote Karl Pearson in 1903, and Herrnstein and Murray fully echo his lament.[9] In their words, "the wrong kind of children are being produced."[10] The country is being overrun by children who share the poor intelligence and sociopathic proclivities of their mostly young, black, and unwed mothers. Left unchecked, this condition may render inevitable the creation of a "custodial state," indeed, a state that will, in Herrnstein and Murray's view, look something like "a high-tech and more lavish version of the Indian reservation" and be administered by those both rich and gifted on behalf of the poor and dull or a "substantial minority of the nation's population."[11]

The Bell Curve restages a tension or contradiction that has plagued liberal capitalist formations throughout their history—that between the ideology of freedom and equality and the social relations and dynamics of power that generate powerlessness and inequalities of status and wealth. Herrnstein and Murray offer as others before them have offered a simple model of social and biological causation that sees hierarchies of advantage and disadvantage as naturally inscribed or genetically driven and maintain, again, as others have, that government cannot "create the equality of condition that nature itself has neglected to produce."[12] The set of arguments they advance and the "evidence" they marshal in support of these arguments, in other words, have enjoyed a long and grim history in the United States—both are tired and well scripted.

Similarly well scripted are the constellation of responses that have greeted Herrnstein and Murray's resuscitation of biologically reductive arguments; I have in mind, specifically, the two anthologies that were published within months of *The Bell Curve: The Bell Curve Debate*, edited by Russell Jacoby and Naomi Glauberman, and *The Bell*

Curve Wars, edited by Steven Fraser.[13] The essays that are gathered in these two rhetorically important and compelling if also predictable collections tend either to take critical aim at the "scientific" pretensions or underpinnings of the *The Bell Curve* or to contest its claims regarding the meaning of the nation's democratic history and egalitarian traditions. On the whole, however, they remain silent with respect to what occupies the good middle third of Herrnstein and Murray's analysis.[14] Indeed, an eerie silence surrounds what I would argue, in the end, ultimately drives their analysis and the eugenically motivated program that grows out of it, notwithstanding the more incendiary issue of IQ: to wit, black women's fertility, reproductive strategies, and out-of-wedlock births. The silence of these collections with respect to black women's fertility and within a popular discourse otherwise exercised by *The Bell Curve*'s claims is significant and consequential. The controversy over *The Bell Curve* forcefully articulates a range of questions having to do with the changing identity of the nation, the existence of something called "IQ," and the still indefinite but possible links between social ills and genetic "errors." What remains uncontested in this debate, however, and what is thus left in place and at play is a set of reasonings and meanings that produces black women's bodies—indeed, the category "black woman"—as the site and source of social pollution and procreative excess, in need of rehabilitation and regulation.

II

I want to begin this section by returning to a claim I made earlier that the primary object of Herrnstein and Murray's ire, the primary subject of their book, and the primary problem they aim to resolve is what they regard as the federally subsidized procreative excesses of self-evidently promiscuous and "dull" black women. What leads me to this strong and, at first glance, implausible reading is an editorial Murray penned in 1993 for the *Wall Street Journal,* the general sentiment of which resurfaces in the only set of substantive policy recommendations *The Bell Curve* authors develop in the concluding chapter of their book. In this editorial, Murray describes illegitimacy as "the single most important social problem of our time," the cause, in his estimation, of crime, drugs, poverty, illiteracy, welfare, and hopelessness. "Single women with children," he maintains, "are a drain on the community's resources and in larger numbers destroy a community's capacity to sustain itself" not only fiscally, but morally, culturally, and, as the arguments of *The Bell Curve* make unmistakably clear, genetically as well.[15]

The views that Murray merely gestures toward in the *Wall Street Journal* essay are more fully developed and lent a genetic basis in *The Bell Curve*. Illegitimacy, in addition to being identified as a business venture, emerges in the book as both a symptom and a consequence of cognitive—which is to say genetic—incapacity. Dull themselves, poor single women produce dull children while also transmitting a delinquent (meaning crime-ridden, drug-driven, poverty-stricken, morally impoverished, welfare-dependent) culture.[16] Dull begets delinquency begets dull begets delinquency, and so it goes at a menacing pace that far surpasses the fertility of citizens who are more cognitively gifted, economically able, socially responsible, and well socialized, indeed, a pace that now jeopardizes both the character and quality of national life and the prospects of national prosperity. To the extent that a remedy exists for checking the depletion of the nation's (cognitive) resources, the remedy lies in implementing policies that alter the relative fertility of each cognitive class and also—ironically, given the biologism of their argument—in fostering adoption. In the final chapter of *The Bell Curve*, "A Place for Everyone," Herrnstein and Murray speak caustically to the question of fertility; I quote them at length:

> Of all the uncomfortable topics we have explored, a pair of the most uncomfortable ones are that a society with a higher mean IQ is also likely to be a society with fewer social ills and brighter economic prospects, and that the most efficient way to raise the IQ of a society is for smarter women to have higher birth rates than duller women. Instead America is going in the opposite direction, and the implication is a future America with more social ills and gloomier economic prospects. These conclusions follow directly from the evidence we have presented at such length, and yet we have so far been silent on what to do about it.
>
> We are silent because we are as apprehensive as most other people about what might happen when a government decides to social engineer who has babies and who doesn't. We can imagine no recommendation for using the government to manipulate fertility that does not have dangers. But this highlights the problem: The United States already has policies that inadvertently social-engineer who has babies, and it is encouraging the wrong women. *If the United States did as much to encourage high-IQ women to have babies as it now does to encourage low-IQ*

women, it would rightly be described as engaging in aggressive manipulation of fertility.

The technically precise description of America's fertility policy is that it subsidizes births among poor women, who are also disproportionately at the low end of the intelligence distribution. We urge generally that these policies, represented by the extensive network of cash and services for low-income women who have babies, be ended. The government should stop subsidizing births to anyone, rich or poor. The other generic recommendation, as close to harmless as any government program we can imagine, is to make it easy for women to make good on their decision not to get pregnant by making available birth control mechanisms that are increasingly flexible, foolproof, inexpensive, and safe.[17]

A "close to harmless" government program that would subsidize birth control for indigent women? The relatively brief legal and legislative history of Norplant in the United States—the birth control clearly alluded to at the end of this passage—suggests that any such program would not be quite the generic benefaction Herrnstein and Murray represent it as being. Approved by the FDA in 1990, Norplant is widely regarded as a flexible, foolproof, relatively reasonable, and inexpensive way—socially, legally, medically, and financially—to induce temporary sterilization. It entails the medical insertion of six capsules in a woman's upper arm and prevents pregnancy for up to five years. At least thirty states thus far have attempted to pass legislation that would make mandatory insertion of the contraceptive a condition for receiving any form of social benefit, and although Medicaid will pay for the insertion of the capsules in many states, it will not also pay for their removal unless their removal is medically indicated.[18] Courts and state legislatures across the country have come increasingly to regard Norplant as the single most practical option for both regulating the fertility of "drug-abusing and violent women"—as women on welfare are frequently described—and "protecting" any current *and unconceived* children they might have.[19] As Michael Rees put the matter in an article for the *New Republic*, "The current threat to children in our inner cities makes [the mandatory insertion of Norplant] an option that the morally serious can no longer dismiss."[20]

Being a single, childbearing woman is what constitutes the mark of deviance and pathology for Herrnstein and Murray, and this is underscored further by their policy prescriptions regarding marriage. In addition to representing temporary sterilization and the termination of all social benefits to unmarried women with children as both "modest and reasonable" ways of interrupting the momentum of the nation's downward spiral, these authors also advocate returning marriage "to its formerly unique status . . . , as the sole legal institution through which rights and responsibilities regarding children are exercised."[21]

> If you are married, you take on obligations. If you are not married, you don't. . . . If you are an unmarried mother, you have no legal basis for demanding that the father of the child provide support. If you are an unmarried father, you have no legal standing regarding the child—not even a right to see the child, let alone any basis honored by society for claiming he or she is "yours."[22]

Finally, in a curious reversal of their argument but as part of their overall policy package, Herrnstein and Murray advocate adoption as the most direct, immediate, and federally inexpensive means for improving a child's cognitive functioning and thus the nation's cognitive resources. "Moving children from a deprived home environment [defined as a single parent, female-headed household] to a very advantaged one appreciably raises cognitive functioning," in their best estimation, by as much as twenty points.[23] It is also, in their words, "cheap." "If the environment matters in bestowing human intelligence,"—and for some purposes, apparently, it does—"we should be able to create extraordinary environments to raise it further."[24]

> Right now, the government has the power to force a parent to give up their children based on evidence of abuse and neglect. While we do not advocate expanding this power, we want to return to the state of affairs that prevailed until the 1960's when children born to single women— where much of the problem of child abuse and neglect originates—were more likely to be given up for adoption.[25]

If, that is, both woman and child happened to be white. Black women tended not to put their out-of-wedlock children up for adoption, although the facts suggest that adoption was simply not an option for most black women in most parts of the country during the period to which Herrnstein and Murray refer. Indeed, "the mandate for a black woman to keep her child was so strong and enforceable that when a black unwed mother tried to put her baby up for adoption in Cook County, Illinois, in the late 1950s, the court charged her with desertion."[26]

But this is to rush the story. I want to pause briefly to consider the magical moment that Herrnstein and Murray invoke in the passage above, to consider, in particular, the resignification of adoption and the meaning of white, nonmarital childbearing in a postwar context of rising rates of "illegitimate" pregnancy among both white and black women. The story is a complicated one, but instructive even if told in the abbreviated and somewhat sparse way that I will tell it here. In this pronatal, profamily postwar 1950s moment, as Ricki Solinger describes it in *Wake Up Little Susie*, there emerges a flourishing and unprecedented market in illegitimate children—a zealous demand for and an earnest recruitment of white babies on the part of infertile middle-class couples eager "for complete family life," defined at the time as including two parents and at least as many children. What accompanies the opening and expansion of this "baby market"—indeed, what both makes it possible and is made possible through it—are shifts in the moral and ontological status of the "illegitimate" white infant and the woman who produces it.[27]

As the Supreme Court's 1927 ruling in *Buck v. Bell* clearly illustrates, out-of-wedlock childbearing and the illicit sex it represents were regarded throughout the 1920s, 1930s, and early 1940s as a symptom and consequence of moral degeneracy and mental incapacity.[28] Both states were considered biological and inheritable and marked a woman's out-of-wedlock offspring as naturally delinquent and defective. In the postwar period and certainly by the end of the 1950s, according to Solinger, this view of unmarried childbearing was tempered at least with respect to white women.[29] During this period, illegitimacy was recast as a mental rather than biological disorder or a symptom of an individual neurosis that could be treated—usually within the walls of a maternity home—arrested, once the woman relinquished her child, and cured, once she married. Putting her (now biologically untainted) infant up for adoption came to be regarded as an act of renunciation and self-denial that functioned not only to redeem a woman morally, but to reestablish her as a worthy female and thus restore her marriageability. "In exchange for their babies," writes Solinger, "white women could reenter normative life."[30] And significantly, those women who refused to give up their infants were identified by social workers, politicians, and psychologists alike as mentally unstable, emotionally unfit, latent homosexuals, and delusional insofar as the "maternal bond" many claimed made it impossible for them to part with their young was said to be possible—as the judge in the Anna Johnson case argued—only in the context of hetero-sexual marriage.[31]

Not surprisingly perhaps, a radically different set of stories and pos-sibilities inhabits and shapes the lives of black women during Herrn-stein and Murray's magical postwar, pre-1960s moment. Indeed, for all intents and purposes, black women were excluded from the institu-tional system and site of rehabilitated "womanhood"—until late in the decade, maternity homes typically took in only white women, and, as I mentioned earlier, black women were expected, in any event, to keep their children (even while they were regarded as mentally and morally deficient for doing so). What needs to be underscored is that the meaning of black women's out-of-wedlock pregnancies was not re-figured during the 1950s; out-of-wedlock childbearing remained the sign of genetic incapacity and of an uninhibited *biological* impulse to copulate and breed.[32] Unlike their white counterparts who enabled in-voluntarily childless couples to form normative families and thus pro-duced a "socially valuable commodity" in the form of adoptable white infants, black women were considered "socially unproductive breed-ers" who produced nothing of value and served no useful social func-tion while depleting social resources. Illegitimacy was read both as evi-dence of their deprived tendencies or lack of maternal nature and as an expression of their antisocial or socially destructive behavior.[33]

III

The picture I have presented of adoption during an era in which the meaning and function of the practice were both significantly refigured, although sketched with admittedly broad strokes, nevertheless pro-vides enough detail to complicate the "modest" recommendation Herrnstein and Murray make that the nation return to a pre-1960s state of affairs with respect to out-of-wedlock childbearing. Notwith-standing the claim that what motivates this recommendation is the possibility of raising an individual's cognitive functioning by as much as twenty points, what seems to me more centrally at stake is the reha-bilitation of the out-of-wedlock pregnant body, indeed, the regulation of the procreating single woman. When viewed through Herrnstein and Murray's pre-1960s lens, the single, procreating female can be nei-ther a "complete woman" nor a "real mother" outside the family and a conventionally sanctioned relationship with a man and, thus, being neither "woman" nor "mother," is truly deviant and dangerous.

The question is, What happens when the procreating body targeted for rehabilitation—the unwed procreating black body—can only resist it, canot *by definition* be rehabilitated, by virtue of being "black," which is to say, by virtue of how the category "black woman" is produced through and signifies within both Herrnstein and Murray's text and the broader cultural context as dull, sexually impulsive, maternally deficient, and parasitic? What happens when "single black woman with child" circulates without interruption within the text and cultural context in opposition to "normative life," indeed, cannot enter or occupy "normative life" because its exclusion as pathology performs the important work of producing and ensuring normativity? And finally, what happens when these meanings are kept in place and at play by the silence of a critical public commentary that otherwise refuses *The Bell Curve*'s more obvious conclusions with respect to intelligence? While clearly rhetorical in part, these questions throw into bold relief what is obvious, dangerous, and potentially deadly about *The Bell Curve*'s arguments and much of the commentary generated in response to them. "What happens" is precisely what is happening: the unwed procreating black body continues to signify as the site of the unrestrained wanton breeding of unwanted babies and as the source of social pollution and pathology. It is by definition incorrigible; by definition, a threat to national prosperity; by definition, in need of containment. Within such a system of signification, "temporary" sterilization in the form of Norplant or Herrnstein and Murray's eugenically motivated proposal comes to appear, as the authors claim it is, a modest, reasonable, and responsible solution where others have failed—indeed, something "the morally serious" across the political spectrum seem increasingly to believe they cannot afford to dismiss.

7 / Replicating the Singular Self: Some Thoughts on Cloning and Cultural Identity

In October 1993, in vitro specialists Jerry Hall and Robert Stillman of George Washington University presented a paper at the annual meeting of the American Fertility Society in Montreal. In this paper, Hall and Stillman provided an account of an experiment they had conducted in which they "cloned" seventeen human embryos, or rather "multiplied them," as *Time* put it, "like the Bible's loaves and fishes into 48."[1] By stripping seventeen two- and three-cell embryos of their outer protective coating, separating these cells, and recoating each with an artificial shell, Hall and Stillman produced forty-eight little genetic units, all of which then commenced to divide, some to the thirty-two-cell stage, or approximately the midway point prior to when an egg would normally attach to the uterine lining. None of the in vitro fertilized embryos were allowed to develop beyond this stage, many self-destructed well before it, and all were discarded after six days.

From all accounts, the experiment itself was of little interest scientifically—embryos are routinely biopsied and "twinned" when preimplantation diagnosis is performed in the case of couples at high risk for genetic disease, and for the past three decades, an assortment of nonhuman species (frogs, cows, goats, sheep, rabbits, and pigs) have been successfully "cloned." Nevertheless, the experiment incited what can only be described as a moment of global hyperventilation. It was denounced by the Japanese Medical Association as "unthinkable" and

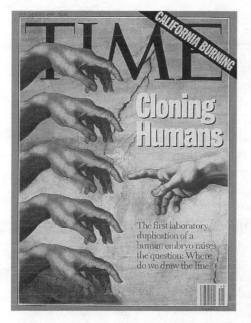

condemned by the Vatican as a practice that "could lead humanity down 'a tunnel of madness.'"[2] German officials reproached the American researchers for their "lack of scruples," noting that such experimentation would be regarded as a criminal offense in Germany, while many French physicians simply dismissed them. As Dr. Jean-François Mattei of Timone Hospital in Marseilles remarked, "This is not research. It's aberrant, showing a lack of a sense of reality and respect for people."[3] Criticized by some in the United States, among them fertility specialists, as marking "a dangerous turn in tampering with life-producing processes," the experiment was also praised by others as one more step along the way toward expanding reproductive choice and thus individual freedom.[4] Indeed, it was this last sentiment that apparently prevailed at the annual meetings where the paper was presented and earned it the conference's first prize.[5]

Notwithstanding the many diverse and impassioned responses to the Hall-Stillman cloning venture, and I will return to consider them in greater detail shortly, there seemed to be a shared sense among the curious, skeptical, and disturbed alike that however preliminary Hall and Stillman's experiment might actually be, it nevertheless traversed and possibly breached some ostensibly fixed, clearly delineated, if also unmarked boundary distinguishing this historical moment as a truly critical juncture, a definitive crossroads, in what is when viewed through a larger historical frame the always ongoing showdown between technoscience and humanism. As one commentator, echoing others, insisted, "There are limits to what human beings ought to be thinking about doing." Indeed, as the less ambivalent but still reticent head of the American Fertility Society asked, "Should this research be done at all?"[6] It is one thing to muck around with the genetic material of livestock or plants to create new or alternative, even hybrid, life forms—this we often call human ingenuity. It is quite another to muck around with the genetic material of humans, particularly in ways that seem to either anticipate or involve modifying, manipulating, or transforming it, which is to say, "us." As *Time*, among other popular newsmagazines, put the matter to and for its readers, "Where do we draw the line?"

In the past three decades, this question has been an almost constant rejoinder to new or imagined reproductive and genetic innovations and the alternative, or perhaps more accurately simply different, forms and practices of life they entail and boldly stage. And it functions, among other ways, as shorthand. It holds the place of a nonexistent moral/public/political discourse—indeed, marks that place with a call instead for a more cogent and comprehensive set of federal guidelines and policies under the auspices of regulatory oversight. It is, in addition, a gesture of control that also signals its absence, for in what sense, either figuratively or literally, can lines of the sort implied be drawn? In what sense is remaking ourselves from the inside out—the possibility raised with cloning, among other biology-based innovations—a question yet to be asked or a set of choices yet to be made? Finally, *Time*'s familiar query in this late-twentieth-century moment of struggle and wonder can be read as a gesture toward fortifying extant borders—in particular those that protect from incursion what is at the same time assiduously patrolled and perpetually produced, the "distinctly human," for example—even as it also marks their realignment. It is, in this regard, a question about identity that assumes and invokes while also signaling a shift in prevailing cultural beliefs about who and what "we" are—indeed, a question whose rhetorical force is largely derived from the transhuman apparitions it typically conjures when posed: the biologically mutant and monstrous who live on the fringes of a frontier just beyond the present (b)order (or line) and who repre-

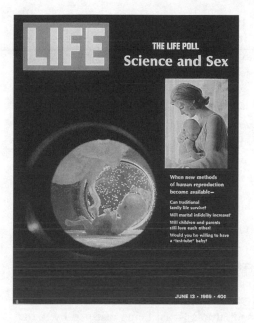

sent, in Leon Kass's words "the end of human life as we and all others know it."[7]

Were we to glance back briefly or situate *Time*'s question in a somewhat broader historical frame, we would find a landscape littered with anxiety and aberration both roaming wild, the imagined effect or concrete embodiment of transgressive crossings.[8] In the late 1960s and early 1970s, for example, when the first tentative steps were taken in the direction of in vitro fertilization, researchers feared and skeptics warned that unrecognizably human creatures would result from scientific interventions in life-producing processes. Theologian Paul Ramsey bitterly welcomed the birth of such monsters, suggesting that only with their birth would such interventions be halted and "authentic humanity" delivered from the threat of immanent erosion and loss. The late Patrick Steptoe, encountered elsewhere in these pages as the "founding father" of in vitro fertilization, moved to allay fears and anxieties about his research in its early phases by reassuring critics that were monstrosities to result from his manipulations of egg and sperm—and he seemed to think they might—no such creatures would be allowed to develop or brought to term.

Similarly, a 1969 issue of *Life* magazine speculated that new reproductive methods would precipitate the dissolution of traditional family life, marital relations, and ties both primordial and social, and give birth to a transhuman entity it called *"in vitro* man."[9] Bearing an uncanny resemblance to Lennon and McCartney's "Nowhere Man," *Life*'s imagined transhuman inhabited what was described as a tissue culture, *post*civilization future. Although technoman might regard himself as happy and "free"—unencumbered by relationship or responsibility and oriented toward play and pleasure—he belongs nowhere and to no one, lives without a sense of place or heritage and, thus, without history. He is, in short and not surprisingly, a mere caricature of his viviparously produced counterpart. Without parents, children, aunts, uncles, and a marriage partner "to whom he [would] owe fidelity," *"in vitro* man" will never be "needed" in precisely the ways *Life* imagined "a man needs to be needed." He lives forever "a stranger and alone" while never recognizing himself as either. And this lack of comprehension renders his predicament, in *Life*'s view, all the more tragic. Finally, in an equally distressed and cautious fashion, *Look* magazine similarly informed its readers in 1971 that "one of mother-nature's most cherished rituals [was] being usurped by man." And *Look*'s vision of the consequences of this appropriation was decidedly dire: "All hell will break loose," it reported, citing Nobel laureate James Watson in a statement Watson made before a congressional committee recommending that Congress move swiftly to outlaw alternative reproductive techniques. "The nature of the bond between parents and children . . . and everyone's values about his individual uniqueness could be changed beyond recognition."[10]

The biologically monstrous, unrecognizably human or transhuman creatures it was feared might be produced by new reproductive and genetic interventions—those on whom transgressive crossings would be visibly inscribed—have not yet materialized. Over the course of the past twenty-five years, these new reproductive and genetic practices have been assimilated into the order of nature or brought into the service of precisely those institutions, relations, and relationships or ways of life they seemed destined to raze, their transgressive potential at least temporarily contained. They are no longer regarded as contrary to the work of nature, but rather as instruments that promote or assist nature's work, enabling, correcting, or improving natural processes that have gone awry and that, in any event, apparently, are highly mercurial and inefficient. In this respect, they are now part of what Sarah Franklin, among others, terms a new "conception narrative," a highly sentimental narrative of biological desire and drive that displaces the image and threat of the technoscientist playing god with portraits of the happy, heterosexual, white nuclear family—dysfunctional, perhaps, but hardly unrecognizable—that would not exist but for "the pioneering efforts of scientists on the frontiers of reproductive discovery."[11]

If monstrosities exist, they are, as the case of Anna Johnson poignantly illustrates, the progeny of legal rather than biological machinations or efforts to track and tell one story of origin, relationship, relatedness, and identity in the voice of the natural when these new practices and processes have rendered such a telling, I am inclined to say "unintelligible," but "afflicted" and "exposed" are perhaps more accurate. As we have seen in each of the essays throughout this book, these new practices have produced a proliferation of possible stories or forms of generation, constellations of relationship, and modes of relatedness that cannot "arise in nature," that transform the meaning of "natural facts" and profoundly refigure what counts as "natural." And in this respect, they have had the effect of destabilizing dominant narratives grounded in nature about who or what is called person, mother, parent, family, fetus, and baby.

At the same time, as we have seen as well, new reproductive practices and processes have also been brought into the service of dominant cultural narratives and work both to facilitate and fortify them, "deploy[ing] very familiar prescriptions under increasingly unfamiliar guises."[12] The rescripting that is required, however, for these new practices to perform such work, to function ideologically, is considerable. And it is at such moments in particular—typically when the law is called upon to locate nature or determine which "natural facts" are "truly" natural and therefore determinant—that the production or, as the law seems generally to view it, "presence" of monsters is made visible. In the context of surrogacy, for example, however one tells the story of the "desperate infertile couple"—and such couples are always represented in popular, legal, and medical discourse as "desperate"— there is still a surplus of bodies, spare parts or figures like Anna Johnson or Mary Beth Whitehead, who are positioned just outside the postpartum frame of the newly fashioned "natural" family unit, at once both integral and extraneous to it. To the extent that they enter the frame or insist on being figured within it, they enter as excess— hosts, receptacles, and foster parents, or delusional, self-serving interlopers whose maternal claims are pathologized and said to jeopardize precisely what their maternal labors have made possible and been solicited to serve.

As in the telling of most genealogical tales, then, where the monstrous was once spied roaming, mothers, fathers, and families now comfortably reside. Notwithstanding the often destabilizing effects of new reproductive practices, these new practices have been domesticated over the course of the past twenty-five years. They are now positioned well within a set of borders—categorical and conceptual, moral and ontological—that, although treated as fixed and given, are clearly only provisional, are themselves in a state of constant fluctuation and realignment, the site, source, and effect of ongoing cultural contests. Returning to *Time*'s proverbial line, where this line seems self-evidently set today and where it was regarded as naturally fixed or drawn a quarter of a century ago are clearly two quite different places. And in this respect, to put the matter in terms of Kass's remonstration, we are, in some sense, always already encountering the end of human life as it is known (or practiced by some). Situated anxiously and precariously on the edge of aberration, we are, in some sense, always already successors to forms and practices of life that circumscribe what is called the distinctly human and seem in danger of giving way for good.

Which returns us to the issue of cloning and the controversy that erupted when Hall and Stillman announced that they had cloned seventeen human embryos. Hall and Stillman presented their experiment as merely the obvious next step in a logical progression that had begun with in vitro fertilization and, thus, properly situated well within a now settled frontier. Once the procedure was technically refined, they suggested, it would simply "boost the efficiency of in vitro" or rather increase the odds of a successful pregnancy by increasing the number of viable embryos available for implantation. Using defective embryos that would never have developed "naturally" or "normally" and that were, in any event, never implanted, the experiment, by their account, was a modest contribution to ongoing global fertility efforts and shared with these efforts the overriding—and, at this point, publicly assumed, accepted, and legitimating—desire to assuage the suffering of infertile couples by expanding the therapies available to them.[13] "I revere human life," Hall is reported to have uttered with choked emotion in response to the public outcry that greeted his research. "We

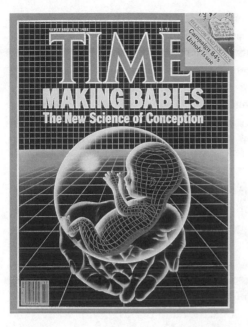

have not created [it] or destroyed [it] in this experiment" but "have set out to provide some basic information."[14]

"Basic information"? When dystopic novels such as *Brave New World* and *1984* constitute an essential part of the civics education of most high school-age youths in the United States and function within contemporary popular discourse on technology, and biology-based technologies in particular, as constitutive tropes, Hall and Stillman's general bewilderment at the public furor and popular flights of fancy their research incited is a bit curious. How could they not have anticipated generating some cultural disturbance? And is their apparently quite genuine bewilderment an expression of the arrogance of the research scientist, or simple naïveté? On the other hand, and more directly at the center of my interest in this chapter in discerning some of the cultural work being done in the context of the controversy over cloning, what is it about the mere prospect of intentionally twinning human life that struck so many as so "unthinkable," that seemed to insult as much as threaten contemporary assumptions, beliefs, and understandings with respect to who and what we are? What precisely is it about an ostensibly contrived genetic "sameness" or an apparent lack of genetic "singularity" that constitutes a "difference" apparently so profound that otherwise intelligent people have wondered whether clones can be considered "legitimate human beings" with a full complement of civil rights and liberties without also noticing the ways in which such considerations reenact the now suspect projects of another age to partialize standards of humanity?[15] What after all is a "legitimate human being," and what is an "illegitimate," "fraudulent," or "counterfeit" one? And in what sense could it be said that the Bill of Rights either presumes or protects genetic purity—or, putting it less provocatively, a "unique" genotype—as the inalienable property of one against the many?

In most respects, the controversy that erupted over the Hall-Stillman cloning venture proffered few surprises. Indeed, in most respects, it was a well-scripted border skirmish in ongoing contests over who and what gets to count as fully human, an occasion for registering anxiety, rehearsing fear, imagining monstrosities, and retelling stories of origin and identity. These stories, at least in the moment of telling, ostensibly reset and settle highly permeable, continuously shifting boundaries that maintain the coherence and exclusivity of what is the ideological centerpiece of Western thought, humanism's unique, self-contained, self-determining individual, assumed and reinforced by as well as produced in and through numerous discursive systems. What most interests me about this skirmish, aside from the way it reiterates many of the same apprehensions that accompanied the introduction of new conceptive technologies in the late 1960s, are the rhetorical strategies that were deployed to rescue humanism's "unique individual," in particular, the appeal to genetics as a self-evident guarantor of individual originality and authenticity as well as cultural diversity. What is curious about the argument from genetics, as we will see, is that it appears to secure "individual identity" at the expense of "autonomy" and "agency" and, thus, to displace what it aims primarily to rescue.[16] While rendering us genetically distinct individuals, in other words, it also, in the end and rather ironically, renders us genetically determined.

The related question of genetics or the geneticization of identity and individuality and cultural diversity is equally as troubled and as troubling, particularly when situated—as I would argue we must, because it is so situated—within a broader social frame and read in relation not only to contemporary mainstream debates about multiculturalism, but to the resurgence of a subtle and not-so-subtle racism that has washed across the country in recent years. For among the more fervent responses to cloning is the charge that it entails the contrived replication and perpetuation into another generation of what already exists and, in (re)producing only sameness, robs the world of the rich heterogeneity that nature—in this case the chance meeting of egg and sperm—would otherwise ensure. It is, of course, the very randomness of nature and the suffering it creates that new reproductive interventions are designed to contain and correct; in fact, "nature's randomness" is precisely what has lent legitimacy to the development of these new technologies in the first place. But, more to the point, even a casual glance across the cultural landscape suggests that far from being richly appreciated, embraced, or encouraged, diversity and difference are often addressed as discrepancy or deviance and, in either case, as problems to be managed.

One could argue, and I will at the risk of seeming once again to be confounding categories and interjecting a politics at precisely the wrong interstice, that social technologies already do much of the work at the same deep level and with the same effect that it is feared this new reproductive technology, cloning, will do and have. Indeed, as each of the controversies reviewed in this book illustrates, the distinction between social technologies and new reproductive ones is formal at best: not only are individuals being reproduced, but so too are the social relations that organize and render them recognizable as such (both to themselves and others). As anthropologist Mary Douglas puts it, "Institutions bestow sameness; they turn the body's shape to their conventions."[17] Sameness, repetition, and replication, in other words, are not the issue, at least not in the terms in which they have been presented as such. The issue, rather, is how to conventionalize and contain diversity and (the proliferation of) difference(s) or how to render diversity and difference socially legible, and this is what geneticizing both would seem in the end, at least ostensibly, to accomplish. What, after all, is the "gene" once mapped now said to promise but a "master code" or "blueprint" that can be deciphered and read?[18] The high anxiety, then, over difference, singularity, and individuality in the context of cloning, coupled with the move to ground and guarantee each in and through genetics, seems to me to hail a pause. For when this anxiety is situated in a larger social frame and considered in terms of a deep-seated and pervasive cultural proclivity to read difference only as threat, a constellation of distortions begins to appear, something like the distortions that emanate from and indicate the presence of a black hole, to borrow an analogy used by Evelynn Hammonds.[19] Although nothing peculiar is obviously in evidence—one would expect a debate about cloning to more or less cluster around precisely the kinds of issues that have in fact been raised—the discursive field, as with the space surrounding black holes, nevertheless seems anomalous, inconstant, unsettled, and curiously warped. This suggests, among other things, that something is present and at play that does not immediately meet the eye.

Before exploring further the insides of this something—or what seem to me to be a confused and rather striking series of displacements, the contours of which I have just briefly sketched—I want to set out in a succinct, but somewhat more systematic, fashion the objections and fears that greeted the Hall-Stillman cloning venture and the prospect of developing a new form and practice of life. These objections more or less cluster around four clearly related sets of issues: the eugenic import of the practice, its potential for (further) commodifying human life, its disruptive effect on "natural" kinship structures, and, finally, its potentially devastating implications with respect to conventional understandings of identity and individuality.

Of these apprehensions, concern surrounding the eugenic possibilities of cloning and other similar practices that work on humans from the inside out is probably the most familiar, most frequently rehearsed, and most thoroughly scripted within the culture. As Diane Paul observes, with respect to the development and application of a wide spectrum of new genetic technologies, "Eugenics [is], in effect, the approved . . . anxiety." Indeed, the specter of eugenics has so thoroughly colonized collective imaginings, fantasies, and critical discourse that a range of otherwise pressing and practical questions are simply eclipsed or ignored. Illustrations of this pervade the literature on biology-based technologies, but consider by way of concrete example, as Paul does, the Human Genome Project: while considerable attention is being directed toward examining the ways in which this project may "open the door" to eugenics—the assumption being that this "door" is not already opened and the passage well trafficked—the less dramatic but absolutely basic question of "whether mapping and sequencing the whole human genome represents a cost-effective way to prevent or cure disease" has for the most part remained formally uninterrogated.[20]

Alongside this question, and others like it, there is the additional problem of determining what precisely "eugenics" now means or entails,[21] notwithstanding what we think we see in images from the 1930s and 1940s or know from novels like *Brave New World* and *1984*. Although the teachings proffered at these sites are compelling, they are obviously not exhaustive and may, in fact, foster a certain myopia with respect to what coercion and domination or a eugenics practice might actually look like in late-twentieth-century North America. Indeed, there are other sites and points of entry that may prove more fruitful than have brave new world scenarios in attempting to discern the shape of eugenics in the context of proliferating "choices" and expanding "freedoms" or practices that are typically said to mark the absence of coercion and domination but may well function as mechanisms of both.

Nevertheless, it was a variety of brave new world scenarios that partially scripted popular responses to the Hall-Stillman cloning venture. The experiment, it was said, marked a critical step in the direction of a world in which master races and subhumans would be genetically engineered, a world in which, as *Time* described it, "cookie cutter humans [would be] baked and bred to order" or, in the words of Jeremy Rifkin, vast armies of identical, "standardized human beings" would be produced according to various specifications.[22] Human/animal hybrids were conjured with horror, as was the possibility—treated widely as the obvious and inevitable outcome of genetic management—that we would soon find ourselves on the verge of creating a socially stratified society, inhabited and divided by different kinds and classes of people. In such a society, "natural" differences would be constitutive of rank or class standing and privilege and would presumably count in ways they currently do not. Indeed, in this society some people would be regarded as more worthy than others and thus as more valuable. Such projected stratification is clearly intended to stand in marked contrast to the world we currently occupy—leaving many of us, then, to speculate about what precisely distinguishes this "vision" of difference from the one proffered by Herrnstein and Murray in *The Bell Curve*. That one is considered horrifying while the other circulates within popular culture as the initiation of a realistic, long-deferred public reckoning is, at best, a curious feat.[23]

If rendering persons mere instruments of some larger social body and design constitutes the nightmare that sits at the center of this first set of objections to cloning, rendering persons mere instruments of another's body and design, producing them for sale or for the sole purpose of harvesting their parts, is the dystopic scenario that organizes the second set of objections. Presented originally in the *New York Times* and later recycled by popular newsmagazines, this account envisions only one of a set of cloned embryos being implanted and brought to term.[24] The other might be put on the market, as gametes now commonly are, its quality (and cost?) appraised in terms of the life trajectory of its twin, or it might be put on ice and "grown" only in the event that its twin dies or needs replacement parts at some later point in life—a heart, lung, kidney, or bone marrow.

These imaginings yield a grim and unsettling vision of an ostensibly alien, unknown, and as yet unmade world—harvesting body parts is the stuff of horror films, after all, and the *National Enquirer,* or an activity periodically ascribed to First World countries by Third World populations to explain what has become a dense international traffic in children, a graphic depiction of colonization, to be sure. But more haunting than the world these scenarios depict is the one they simply ignore. One need not stage an encounter with a grim, unruly future to grasp the set of effects produced when bodies are rendered commodified technologies, objects of commerce, or instruments of another's will, right, desire, and design: such is the still only partially grasped legacy of slavery that continues to figure and frame the meaning and management of the reproductive black body.[25] But alongside this legacy and more than incidentally related to it is an expanding collection of contemporary controversies that reflect a mixture of profound confusion and doubt with respect to what constitutes such practices as bodily integrity and self-sovereignty or what it means to own and have property in the body (and its parts).

Recall, for a moment, the 1991 case of a couple who decided to reproduce for the sole purpose of providing a compatible bone marrow donor for their teenage daughter when no donor could be found and who candidly acknowledged that they did not desire more children and would not have elected to have more were their daughter not in need.[26] Or, to give these same issues a somewhat different inflection, consider as well the 1984 case of John Moore, a leukemia patient whose blood was used without his knowledge or explicit consent to develop the patented and commercially lucrative "Mo Cell Line."[27] Was Moore's "interest" in his body parts waived when he signed a general consent form authorizing UCLA's Pathology Department to remove and dispose of his organs? In what sense and under what conditions are body parts property (commodities) and alienable (available for sale)? Consider from yet another sphere of controversy the confused and troubled thinking that has surrounded the harvesting of ovum, brain tissue, and assorted other materials from aborted fetuses. These examples together suggest that the "ethical" questions Hall and Stillman by their own account sought to "get moving" by cloning human embryos are clearly already at play within the culture and obviously not only or simply with respect to biomedical innovations and interventions:[28] the body as material resource is hardly an issue peculiar to cloning, although cloning may bring this issue into particularly sharp relief. But also clearly at play are new and disowned forms and practices of life whose operation and effects are fundamentally refiguring present forms and practices, conspicuously altering and thereby postponing the very future in which they are nevertheless thought to be situated and considered a menacing and, as yet, unrealized part.

The third cluster of anxieties voiced in response to cloning and the Hall-Stillman experiment merely underscores this point or works, similarly, to pull our gaze back from a dreamscape of dark imaginings to see in present practices and processes precisely those apocalyptic elsewheres that supposedly belong to some dim future world just beyond *Time*'s proverbial line. At the center of this third set of hesitations is the charge that cloning would disrupt what appears to be an irreversible, linear sequencing of generations, thereby disassembling a kinship structure that is conventionally regarded not as a social or discursive technology, but as a "natural" and naturally ordered set of arrangements and relationships. The natural progression or descent of generations, each adding something new and unique to the entire "stock," thereby guaranteeing diversity, would give way with cloning, or so it is feared, to a contrived perpetuation of what already exists.[29] Twins could be separated by years or decades, thus robbing the second born of an original, unlived life of its own.[30] More disturbing still, for some, is the possibility that who we call "mother" we could also call "sister." What happens to conventional understandings of familial relationships and, in particular, the "parent-child bond," or conventional prohibitions with respect to incest when parent and child can potentially be not just siblings, but twins separated by decades?

Although lines of descent have yet to be breached in precisely this way, over the past several years embryo transfers have produced curious generational mixings: birth mothers have simultaneously become grandmothers with delivery. Postmortem ventilation therapies, as we saw in chapter 2, and instances in which conception was accomplished with sperm obtained upon the death of a "parent" similarly work to confuse, complicate, and challenge conventional assumptions with respect to generational succession, by obscuring, for example, the boundary between (as well as the meaning of) what is called living and dead.[31] Finally, suspending the development of simultaneously conceived in vitro embryos—implanting some while freezing others—is now a fairly routine practice that potentially poses precisely the situation foregrounded by objections to cloning, that of twins being born years or lifetimes apart, with one, apparently significant, difference: twins produced in this fashion are not "identical." Even while their separation in years may be contrived, in other words, each nevertheless retains its genotypic integrity, which is to say—speaking now in the register of popular discourse—a singular and original "self." Neither usurps the life or identity of the other through replication—indeed, as Arthur Caplan puts it, neither is potentially forced to see in the figure of its double "something about [its] future that [it] do[esn't] want to see."[32]

Each of the three sets of objections briefly considered thus far—the concern for the eugenic import of cloning, its potential for further commodifying human life, and its disruptive effect on natural kinship structures—clearly implicate questions of identity and individuality. Notwithstanding their somewhat different points of focus, all three work to stage and contain the insult that intentionally twinning human life seems self-evidently to pose to conventional beliefs, understandings, and assumptions regarding who and what we are. Questions of identity and individuality are, nevertheless, explicitly articulated in the context of the cloning controversy and constitute what I want to take up as the fourth and final, most impassioned, set of hesitations greeting the Hall-Stillman effort. Grounded in appeals both to law and genetics and registering a deep skepticism at the prospect of producing life forms that appear to lack a singular, hence authentic, well-bounded, naturally given "self," these hesitations traverse what is a rather predictable if also colorful terrain. Daniel Callahan of the Hastings Institute, for example, put the matter this way for Gina Kolata of the *New York Times*: "We have a right to our own individual genetic identity. I think this will violate that right."[33] Reiterating Calla-

han's concern, but shifting its emphasis to foreground what is a culturally pervasive anxiety over the shared and the singular—the "more" of
some one thing not being in any sense "merrier"—Arthur Caplan, di-
rector of the Center for Bioethics at the University of Minnesota, had
this to say, again for the *Times*: "One of the things that we treasure
about ourselves is our individuality. When you deliberately set out to
make copies of something, you lessen its worth."[34] Finally, transfixed
by the image of an otherwise indivisible self fracturing at the hands of
technoscientists, Germain Grisez, professor of Christian ethics at
Mount St. Mary's College, called upon researchers to place themselves
in the same position they were considering placing others. In Grisez's
words, "The people doing this ought to contemplate splitting themselves in half and see how they like it."[35]

The individual conjured in these renderings, and in the cloning controversy more generally, is clearly not regarded as either a function of
ideology or a relatively recent accomplishment of particular discipli-
nary practices that took hold in the seventeenth and eighteenth cen-
turies. Nor is this individual seen, moreover, as a historical formation,
the product of various discursive strategies and institutionalized discourses, a social technology, or even, for that matter, a social creature
in any meaningful sense of the word *social*. The individual of the
cloning controversy emerges rather as a self-evident fact of nature or a
fixed, stable, noncontingent value. It is an utterly nonrelational entity,
indeed, an entity whose definitive features—whose individuality, authenticity, unique difference, or thoroughly contained and autonomous self—are regarded as genetically inscribed, guaranteed, and
given properties, the potential theft or (unauthorized) appropriation
of which may now require policing.[36]

As it happens, we have encountered this entity elsewhere in these
pages in the context of other controversies. Recall part of the court's
reasoning in the Anna J. case, for example, its invocation of genetics to
establish the identity of the fetus Johnson gestated and, thus, settle the
question of precisely whose product and property the fetus actually
was. Drawing on the testimony of UC Irvine child psychologist and
pediatrician Dr. Justin David Call, the court argued that who and
what the fetus was and would become—its individual genealogical,
physiological, and psychological identity—had already been determined genetically. Its "outcome" had more or less been fixed by its
genes, and this, in the judge's view, gave the child's genetic contribu-

tors the greater claim to its rearing. What appears to have escaped the court's notice, however—the irony of its decision, as ethicist George Annas observes—is that the same overt reasoning used to grant the Calverts custody could have similarly been deployed to sustain quite the opposite conclusion. As Annas explains, "If genetics determines 70 percent of our IQ and most of our psychological make-up regardless of the type of home environment we are raised in within Western middle-class society, then it becomes very difficult to make a 'best interests' of the child argument for rearing by the genetic parents. The child will as likely do as well with *any* parents, because the child's genes, rather than the environment, will determine its future."[37]

If the Anna J. case is one site where we have already encountered the radically self-contained, self-producing, ostensibly original individual of the cloning controversy, the debate about abortion and, in particular, the production of the "fetus as person" is another site. Although we have traversed this terrain in considerable detail elsewhere, it nevertheless seems useful to return to it briefly and note that in an emerging medical literature shaped by what is called the new science of fetology and current genetic research now directed toward discerning not merely the "facts of life" but the "secrets of life,"[38] a curious story of origins, agency, and individuality is being produced that features the fetus as a self-made liberal subject in utero. Considered once a passive and parasitic passenger, the fetus has come increasingly to be represented in both medical and scientific literatures as the "dominant, active partner in pregnancy,"[39] autonomous, self-regarding, and more or less self-sufficient, aware of its own interests from conception, apparently, and capable of acting upon these interests. As one physician describes it, the fetus is "an egoist [rather than] a helpless dependent . . . [whose] purpose is to see that its own needs are met."[40] Its genetic blueprint is now said to establish its unique identity, regulate its developmental direction, and settle the parameters of its future achievement(s). Indeed, its genetic blueprint "starts its clock," supplies its purpose, and, paraphrasing Franklin, distinguishes the fetus as the principal architect of its own miraculous transformation.[41]

This portrait of the "self-made individual/fetus" proffers a clear if confused rendering of at least one version of the liberal story. It geneticizes what C. B. MacPherson has dubbed the "possessive individual," inscribes as raw biology liberal understandings of self-ownership and interest, and reinvigorates a masculinist fantasy of autonomy, agency, and control that rivals even the more radical ruminations of early liberal thinkers insofar as these were constrained by some sense of the divine (however anemic). If human beings exist as distinct and preformed individuals prior to any social bonds, proprietors of their own attributes and capacities, by virtue of some genetic code, and if their singular existence—or what, in the context of the cloning controversy, is called "the self"—is solely or principally a "coded" and thus closed matter, a matter of genetic material fixed by nature and pregiven, perhaps it makes sense to talk about guaranteeing someone a right to their own genetic identity, as Callahan puts it. However, we might first want to consider precisely what is being guaranteed and to whom (or what). Do we really mean to reduce identity—or this thing that is being called "the self"—to genetic patterns or strands of a few basic chemicals the complex sequencing and functioning of which we have only the most modest understanding?[42] In what sense, exactly, are these chemicals or, perhaps more accurately, their effect what we would call a "person," an "individual," or a "self"? By the same token, what does it mean to geneticize or read back to the gene liberalism's atomistic and apprehensive understanding of individuals? What precisely is solved by characterizing the fetus as a more or less self-sufficient, utterly self-regarding, radically self-interested, nonrelational agent—a thoroughly masculinized entity with an independent will, indeed, an "egoist" who "induces changes in maternal physiology" in order to render its "host" suitable and who is engaged in what can, at best, be described as a thoroughly instrumental, parasitic relationship?[43] And, finally, in what ways does it even make sense to talk about "agency," "control," and "autonomy" when the "distinct self" is itself genetically determined?

Rescuing humanism's unique, radically contained, and separate individual by an appeal to nature in the form of genetics works, at least rhetorically, to preserve the idea of originality, authenticity, indivisibility, and natural diversity. It also reinstalls a creature that bears a convincing likeness to the one potentially displaced by cloning, certainly a creature that is still more or less coherent within dominant discursive systems and can (continue to) be assimilated and accounted for by them, at least superficially. In the process of being discursively reassembled as a thoroughly geneticized entity, however, this creature has undergone a slight but significant transmogrification. In other words, although genetic essentialism may allow for the recuperation of "singularity," it also profoundly complicates what are conventionally regarded as other equally integral or constitutive aspects of identity—conventional notions of agency and responsibility, for example, or freedom and autonomy. These practices presume a rational, unified, sovereign subject, in control and fully accountable. To accommodate an understanding of individuals as essentially driven or constrained by particular genetic traits or the legacy of a particular genetic history, they cannot be simply transposed or expanded, but would need, instead, to be radically refigured.[44] Without such a refiguration, genetically given difference can signify only—as it currently often does—as individual pathology: deficiency, disorder, and deviance. Within the context of conventional understandings of "agency," "responsibility," "freedom," and "autonomy," such difference will operate only to reinscribe and enforce a normative map of the "distinctly" or fully human—operate, in other words, as a means for organizing and regulating certain kinds of persons and classes of people.[45]

Perhaps the more significant if obvious point, however, is that genetics is itself a rich and protean medium for ventriloquy: it is hardly an uncanny coincidence that liberalism's particular understandings and organization of "self," indeed, a liberal political order not to mention particular kinship practices—all of which are historically recent, highly contingent formations—are precisely what modest decodings of the molecular text seem now to suggest are genetically inscribed. In and of themselves, genes have no transparently meaningful or socially significant stories to tell that researchers simply discern or transcribe; they contain no intrinsic or self-evident social truths, and suggest, explain, guarantee, prescribe, predict, codify, confirm, and document nothing. To the degree that they have explanatory power of the sort invoked and appealed to in the cloning controversy, for example, or the case of Anna Johnson, or the debate about abortion, that power is clearly derivative and contextual.

Animated by a rich and resilient constellation of ideological narratives, genes function within culture and within the body in culture as condensed arguments and contests: they are one way of explaining the world and our place in it in an ostensibly disinterested or objective fashion. They are as well a way of talking about social relations and relationships that places both beyond the scope of argument, preserves extant social arrangements, and casts social interventions of the sort promoted by the now widely ridiculed Great Society programs of the

1960s as ineffective and destabilizing. Finally, genes function within culture and within the body in culture as a way of ordering and organizing difference and identity that detaches both from any field of purpose.

A good illustration of this is, again, the Anna J. case, when the judge located the deep roots of identity and enduring ties in genetics and argued that the child Christopher's sense of "selfhood" would be imperiled were he either reared by Johnson, "a genetic hereditary stranger," rather than by those with whom he shares a genetic history, or raised in the context of a three-parent, two-mom kinship group—a situation, as we saw, that he described as "ripe for crazy-making." This familial arrangement is certainly one that confounds extant law and troubles extant social relations and beliefs. And, to be sure, contemporary racialized practices of difference and contemporary configurations and practices of kinship and identity—or the prevailing structure(s) of our social lives—lend force to the judge's assessment of the conditions most likely to produce or disable something resembling a conventionally recognizable and coherent sense of self. But, to cite Mary Douglas again, an institution—in this case the law—bestows sameness: "It compels things to be as it recognizes they are." As even the most cursory historical or cross-cultural overview suggests, there is nothing biologically "inevitable" about the singular self or the two-parent, heterosexual family unit that is one among many institutions charged with its replication. Different social formations clearly engender different life forms, or, to put this same matter somewhat differently, following legal scholar Katharine Bartlett, "Although we pretend otherwise, it seems clear that our judgements about what is best for children are as much the result of social and political judgements about what kind of society we prefer as they are conclusions based upon neutral or scientific data."[46]

Ontological productions are densely orchestrated, ongoing cultural reproductions—they are about the reproduction of a particular life form and particular forms of life. Such (re)productions are not, as the judge in the Anna J. case or, for that matter, popular discourse in the context of the cloning controversy seems to suggest, about genetic mandates, even though both nature and genetics may be deployed as grounding alibis that explain, contain, and, of course, authorize and sanction them.[47] Indeed, with respect to cloning, although appeals are made to genetic essentialism to account for and preserve the singular,

indivisible self against the onslaught of practices that threaten its production, genetic essentialism is itself a production of "self" that devi-
ates in significant ways, at least *in effect*, from dominant renderings.
Although invoked to preserve one kind of creature, genetic essentialism discursively refigures what it allegedly reveals as fixed, *in effect*
producing another.

At the outset of this chapter, I suggested that the cloning controversy
was a well-scripted border skirmish. I meant to imply by this that the
controversy functioned to reset what are highly permeable, continuously shifting boundaries that circumscribe the distinctly human.
Through the specter of what "human" might become if these boundaries are transgressed or effaced, humanism's unique, self-contained,
self-determining individual is recuperated at least rhetorically—
another insult and potential onslaught ostensibly, certainly discursively, countered and contained.

Worth noticing in the skirmish over cloning—as well as in each of
the other controversies examined in this book—are the subtle and significant ways in which the meanings and practices that constitute this
entity are being refigured. These changes are, for the most part, ob-
scured by the more spectacular images of monstrosity that are paraded
across the cultural landscape, capturing our attention for the moment,
but, in the end, inciting relief more than fear. They seem, in fact, to deliver us from fear, for notwithstanding the fleeting doubts or hesitations that call these monsters forth when borders are disturbed or conventional social arrangements and relations are disrupted—as they are
continuously—it seems clear that we are neither the subhuman creatures nor the transhuman caricatures each age imagines the next will
or could become. In spite of—and, perhaps, ironically because of—the
proliferation of new reproductive practices and processes, we are still
apparently recognizable to ourselves. The specter of "*in vitro* man"
has long since been displaced—or rather domesticated—by images of
the desperately infertile, but, more than this, as we have seen, many of
the issues that congeal around cloning or seem uniquely staged by the
mere prospect of this and other novel reproductive practices circulate
within the culture in considerably less spectacular and apparently less
pressing forms. The border over which cloning intensifies reflection, in
other words, is hardly untrafficked territory.

Having said this, it is also the case that one cannot track ongoing,
and sometimes seismic, shifts in the landscape of contemporary repro-

ductive practices and politics without, at times, experiencing a sense of vertigo and apprehension. Some combination of both is registered at points in this chapter and each of the previous ones, but not in response to the imagined loss of a transhistorical, authentic, humanity, the loss of a transcendent subject who can only suffer the changes wrought by technoscience, or to what some have argued is a well-organized conspiracy among antifeminist "reproductive engineers" to appropriate women's procreative capacities.[48] Each of these readings, among other similar kinds, produces a morally and politically circumscribed, if also predictable, map that is of little use in the end for navigating the constellations of often contradictory meanings that are generated by and deployed to make sense of new reproductive practices and processes in this late-twentieth-century moment. The apprehension that is discernible throughout this book emerges, rather, in response to the often reactionary, racialized, class-based, and gendered scriptings that both organize the public meaning(s) of these new practices and their proliferating excesses and are being reauthored and authorized through them in the courts, clinics, and culture at large.

Ethicist Albert Johnson speculated in an article that appeared in the *New York Times* following the announcement of the Hall-Stillman experiment that "the first attempts to clone [would] leave us with the possibility [of] creat[ing] a lot of monsters."[49] He went on to suggest, however, that once the procedure is technically refined, the possibility of monstrosity will diminish. In the process of settling the many discursive confusions and contests that have accompanied new reproductive and genetic techniques and their gradual (and ongoing) assimilation into the order of things as instruments that enable nature rather than presage its end, monsters have indeed been created and contained. These perceived monstrosities include the former sex-worker surrogate Mary Beth Whitehead, the gestational surrogate Anna Johnson, and the black, otherwise unidentified, woman—described in the press only as a "Third World citizen"—who was widely denounced when it was learned that she had been implanted with eggs from a white donor, *at her request*, so that her offspring might escape racial discrimination. Additionally construed publicly as among the monstrous is the always unfit and black welfare-dependent single mother, whose fertility—with the advent of Norplant—may now be the price of her freedom; the pregnant woman who smokes, drinks, or otherwise engages in activities that are considered potentially detrimental to fetal life; and, finally, the retired woman who avails herself of post-menopausal therapies and whose successful pregnancy is derisively characterized as "Frankensteinian" and internationally condemned as an aberration of nature.

These are clearly not the kinds of monsters that Johnson or those who greeted incipient in vitro fertilization procedures twenty-five years ago have or had in mind. They are, nevertheless, the monsters that emerge when extant borders, categories, identities, and relations are breached and whose very presence or production permits these borders to regain their coherence and exclusivity. Similar kinds of monsters will undoubtedly be produced and contained in the context of contests over cloning and will likewise perform the important cultural function of securing what the practice destabilizes. Such monsters signify an excess of cultural meaning, are hybrids of meaning—are, simultaneously, both problem and possibility. Their proliferation is necessary and inevitable and suggests that the issue with respect to the panoply of new reproductive practices and processes is not whether these new practices are good or bad; following Marilyn Strathern's eloquent framing of the matter in an altogether different register, the issue, in the end, is rather "how we should think them and how they will think us."

Notes

Introduction

1. In areas where abortion services are unavailable, women seeking abortion are typically forced to travel across state lines for health services. At the particular clinic in question, 20 to 30 percent of the clientele consisted of out-of-state travelers.

2. *Bray v. Alexandria Women's Health Clinic*, 113 S.Ct. 753 (1993), 13.

3. Ibid., 15.

4. Ibid., 12.

5. Ibid., 13.

6. Ibid. (Stevens's dissent with Blackmun concurring), 51–53.

7. There is subtle shift worth noting with respect to how abortion is being read/configured in this dissent. In *Roe v. Wade*, abortion is defined as first and foremost a medical matter and the purview of medical professionals. In *Bray*, Stevens characterizes abortion—and apparently Blackmun accepts the characterization—as a distinctly female practice or a practice in which only women engage. Clearly the discourse on fetal life has forced a refiguring that foregrounds women.

8. What is at issue here is what kind of right abortion is. See *Bray*, 54–55 of Stevens's dissent.

9. For some of the ways in which these issues have been figured in legal discourse, see Reva Siegel, "Reasoning from the Body: A Historical Perspective on Abortion Regulation and Questions of Equal Protection," *Stanford Law Review* 44 (1992): 261–381.

10. Quoted in Peggy Phalen, *Unmarked: The Politics of Performance* (New York: Routledge, 1993), 143: "What has happened to the women's movement?" the organization's newsletter, *Rescue Report*, asked in a 1990 editorial: "We have picked it up; we have become the true defenders of women in this generation by allowing women to be what God intended them to be. We are the ones who are intervening for women in the courts. We are the ones helping single women raise their families." In this passage the discursive terrain occupied by feminists is appropriated and reinflected to produce a

133

world not unlike the one to which the women's movement of the mid-1960s rose up in response. It is a world in which women are regarded as helpless (in need of defense), vulnerable (in need of protection), powerless (in need of refuge), and "allowed" or expected to subordinate all aspects of their lives to their primary, divinely ordained purpose or natural function, the bearing and rearing of children. What Operation Rescue represents as its "feminist turn," in other words, is an innate maternalism, paternalistically rendered, or a not-so-new variation, clearly, on an old and tired tune. It recasts women who seek abortions as helpless victims in need of protection and support and incapable of making such decisions for themselves while valorizing the deeds of the "born-again male hero" or "man-father-Father figure." He acts on their behalf, for their sake, in their best interest, and one could presume, given the logic of paternalism, to check their (mistaken) convictions when necessary in order to "save [them] as well as [their] babies from the capacious maw of death." Susan Harding, "If I Should Die before I Wake: Jerry Falwell's Pro-Life Gospel," in *Uncertain Terms: Negotiating Gender in American Culture*, ed. Faye D. Ginsberg and Anna Lowenhaupt Tsing (Boston: Beacon, 1990), 81.

A benevolent paternalism might be preferred to and certainly has greater popular appeal than a more punishing variety that condemns women who seek abortions as selfish, sinful, murderous, and dangerously unnatural—this was the view of women that Operation Rescue espoused prior to its "feminist" conversion. Paternalism may also seem neither aberrant nor irrational, but perfectly consistent within still-prevalent social and dominant legal understandings that see who and what women are and are for as physiologically rooted and determined. As legal scholar Reva Siegel observes, "Facts about women's bodies [or what Siegel refers to as physiological naturalism], have long served to justify regulation enforcing judgements about women's roles[, alleged needs, assumed wants, and supposed desires]." "Reasoning from the Body," 277. In either case, however, whether benevolent or punitive, respectable or aberrant, Operation Rescue's paternalism and the innate maternalism for which its "feminism" functions as a cover story would seem nevertheless to betray and perpetuate precisely what the majority opinion in *Bray* dismissed as erroneous: a basic attitude or animus toward women, indeed, a derogatory view of women that the record clearly shows could work and has worked, historically, in invidiously discriminatory or exclusionary ways.

11. W. J. T. Mitchell, *Iconology: Image, Text, Ideology* (Chicago: University of Chicago Press, 1986), 38.

12. O'Connor in *Akron*, quoted in David J. Garrow, *Liberty and Sexuality: The Right to Privacy and the Making of Roe v. Wade* (New York: Macmillan, 1994), 643–44.

13. See, for example, Mary Lyndon Shanley, "'Surrogate Mothering' and Women's Freedom: A Critique of Contracts for Human Reproduction," *Signs* 18 (1993): 618–38; Carole Pateman, *The Sexual Contract* (Stanford, Calif.: Stanford University Press, 1988), 209–18.

14. For a good survey of this terrain, see Larry Gostin, ed., *Surrogate Motherhood: Politics and Privacy* (Bloomington: Indiana University Press, 1990).

15. In "traditional surrogacy," the surrogate contributes genetic material, an egg; in gestational surrogacy, the surrogate makes no genetic contribution.

16. "It's interesting in a way, when you relate that [hiring someone to 'carry your child'] back to a practice that went on far into this century of women of means hiring young girls from the village to serve as wetnurses, and often times motherhood ended at birth as far as the work side of it, and I'm not sure anyone would argue that the person that nursed the child for a year from 7lbs to 30lbs got parental rights and became the

mother. It would be interesting to study the bonding psychology. . . . in those situations. There may still be wetnurses today, I don't know. Anyway, I digressed." Indeed. Trial transcript, *Johnson v. Calvert,* Office of the Supreme Court, California (1990), 1495.

17. Sarah Franklin, "Romancing the Helix: Nature and Scientific Discovery," *Romancing Revisited,* ed. L. Pearce and J. Stacey (London: Falmer, 1995).

18. Charles Murray, "The Coming White Underclass," *Wall Street Journal,* October 29, 1993, A14. See also Murray's "Stop Favoring Unwed Mothers," *New York Times,* January 16, 1992, A23: "The problem is not that single mothers are on welfare, but that there are so many single mothers concentrated in poor communities. . . . The single-parent family does not work very well, even under the best of circumstances. . . . Children learn to be responsible adults by watching what responsible adults do. The absence of such examples for young men is especially dangerous. The violence and social chaos in the inner cities show us what happens when about half a generation of males is born to single women.

"The solution lies neither in social programs nor in making women on welfare go to work. It lies in restoring a situation in which almost all women either get pregnant after they get married or get married after they get pregnant. . . . Communities did not need lessons in how to bring these things about until welfare took over. But, to revitalize the natural mechanisms that used to work so effectively we have to come to terms with a fact that is unfashionable to acknowledge and palpably inequitable. For whatever complicated reasons—not least, because women bear children—communities have much more leverage over the woman's behavior than the man's."

19. Mary Douglas, *How Institutions Think* (Syracuse: Syracuse University Press, 1986), 63, 92.

1 / Impaired Sight or Partial Vision?
Tracking Reproductive Bodies

1. Oliver Sacks, "To See and Not See," *New Yorker,* May 10, 1993, 59.

2. Ibid.

3. Ibid., 61.

4. Ibid.

5. Ibid.

6. Ibid.

7. Ibid, 65.

8. Ibid., 70.

9. Donna Haraway, "Situated Knowledges: The Science Question in Feminism and the Privilege of Partial Perspective," in *Simians, Cyborgs, and Women: The Reinvention of Nature* (New York: Routledge, 1991), 190. For fuller discussion of these and related issues, see W. J. T. Mitchell, *Iconology: Image, Text, Ideology* (Chicago: University of Chicago Press, 1986); Jonathan Crary, *Techniques of the Observer: On Vision and Modernity in the Nineteenth Century* (Cambridge: MIT Press, 1995); Lorraine Daston and Peter Galison, "The Image of Objectivity," *Representations* 40 (1992): 81–128.

10. Kimberlé Crenshaw and Gary Peller, "Reel Time/Real Justice," *Reading Rodney King, Reading Urban Uprising,* ed. Robert Gooding-Williams (New York: Routledge, 1993), 57–58.

11. This reversal is set out and critically examined in Judith Butler's masterful essay, "Endangered/Endangering: Schematic Racism and White Paranoia," in *Reading Rod-*

ney King, Reading Urban Uprising, ed. Robert Gooding-Williams (New York: Routledge, 1993), 15–22.

12. The Rodney King video was not the first tape of its kind. Frustrated by the lack of institutional response to community charges and testimony of police abuse, activists in Los Angeles had pursued the strategy, prior to the King beating, of distributing video cameras in communities where excessive force and harassment were routine, in the hopes of establishing some kind of objective record that might then bolster claims of abuse in court. Much of the footage that *Inside Edition* and its brethren showed following the Rodney King incident of police violence was edited from tapes collected by these activists. What is truly curious is that the very existence of this additional footage and what it suggested with respect to the King incident went unremarked. Didn't anyone wonder how a show like *Inside Edition* was suddenly able to air such footage or, for that matter, question what it meant that, aware of its existence and having access to it, they hadn't aired it sooner?

13. Crenshaw and Peller, "Reel Time," 58–59.

14. Robert Gooding-Williams, "'Look a Negro!'" in *Reading Rodney King, Reading Urban Uprising*, ed. Robert Gooding-Williams (New York: Routledge, 1993), 166.

15. Crenshaw and Peller, "Reel Time," 59.

16. Gooding-Williams, "'Look a Negro!'" 167. See also Dagmar Barnouw, "Seeing and Believing: The Thin Blue Line of Documentary Objectivity," *Common Knowledge* 4, no. 1 (1995): 129–43.

17. Haraway, "Situated Knowledges," 188.

18. Gooding-Williams, "'Look a Negro!'" 166. Crenshaw and Peller make a similar point; "Reel Time," 66–67.

19. Patricia J. Williams, "Hate Radio: Why We Need to Tune In to Limbaugh and Stern," *Ms.*, March/April 1994, 26.

20. Gooding-Williams, "'Look a Negro!'" 166.

21. See Sarah Franklin, "Postmodern Procreation: A Cultural Account of Assisted Reproduction," in *Conceiving the New World Order: The Global Politics of Reproduction*, ed. Faye D. Ginsberg and Rayna Rapp (Berkeley: University of California Press, 1995); Sarah Franklin, "Deconstructing 'Desperateness': The Social Construction of Infertility in Popular Representations of New Reproductive Technologies," in *The New Reproductive Technologies*, ed. Maureen McNeil, Ian Varcoe, and Steven Yearly (London: Macmillan, 1990).

22. Janet L. Dolgin, "Family Law and the Facts of Family," unpublished manuscript (1992), 34. This work appeared subsequently as "Just a Gene: Judicial Assumptions about Parenthood," *UCLA Law Review* 40 (1993): 637–94. See also the trial transcript, *Johnson v. Calvert*, Office of the Supreme Court, California (1990), 1490.

23. Trial transcript, *Johnson v. Calvert*, 1487.

24. Alternative family formations were recommended in the Johnson case. See ACLU briefs citing cross-cultural kinship practices and urging the court to adopt a wider lens in fashioning the kinship unit in this case: brief amicus curiae of the American Civil Liberties Union of Southern California, Jon W. Davidson and Paul L. Hoffman (August 1991); brief amicus curiae of the American Civil Liberties Union of Southern California, Jon W. Davidson, Carol A. Sobel, and Paul Hoffman (December 1992).

25. Steven Mason, *A History of the Sciences* (New York: Collier, 1968); see also Aristotle, *Generation of Animals*, trans. A. L. Peck (Cambridge: Harvard University Press, 1979).

26. Londa Schiebinger, *The Mind Has No Sex? Women in the Origins of Modern*

Science (Cambridge: Harvard University Press, 1989), 203, 209; see chap. 7 especially for a more lengthy account.

27. Stephen Jay Gould, *The Mismeasure of Man* (New York: Norton, 1981). See also Cynthia Eagle Russett, *Sexual Science: The Victorian Construction of Womanhood* (Cambridge: Harvard University Press, 1989).

28. Gould, *The Mismeasure of Man*, 54. Londa Schiebinger offers a reading on the issue of fraud in science quite similar to Gould's in *The Mind Has No Sex?* 206–13.

29. Donna Haraway, "Investment Strategies for the Evolving Portfolio of Primate Females," in *Body/Politics: Women and the Discourses of Science*, ed. Mary Jacobus, Evelyn Fox Keller, and Sally Shuttleworth (New York: Routledge, 1990), 148. See also Thomas Laqueur, *Making Sex: Body and Gender from the Greeks to Freud* (Cambridge: Harvard University Press, 1990), chap. 1.

30. For an evenhanded assessment of contemporary research aimed at identifying the biological basis for sex and gender differences, see Helen E. Longino, *Science as Social Knowledge: Values and Objectivity in Scientific Inquiry* (Princeton, N.J.: Princeton University Press, 1990), especially chaps. 6–8.

31. James D. Goldberg, "Introduction,"in "Fetal Medicine" (special issue), ed. James D. Goldberg, *Western Journal of Medicine* 159 (1993): 259.

32. Michael R. Harrison et al., "Fetal Treatment 1982," *New England Journal of Medicine* 307 (1982): 1651–52, quoted in Ruth Hubbard, *The Politics of Women's Biology* (New Brunswick, N.J.: Rutgers University Press, 1992), 175.

33. W. Beard and P. W. Nathanielsz, eds., *Fetal Physiology and Medicine* (London: W. B. Saunders, 1976), v, cited in Sarah Franklin, "Fetal Fascinations: New Dimensions to the Medical-Scientific Construction of Fetal Personhood," in *Off Centre: Feminism and Cultural Studies*, ed. Sarah Franklin, Celia Lury, and Jackie Stacey (New York: HarperCollins, 1991), 192.

34. Michael R. Harrison, "Fetal Surgery," in "Fetal Medicine" (special issue), ed. James D. Goldberg, *Western Journal of Medicine* 159 (1993): 341.

35. Frederic Frigoletto, quoted in Lucy H. Labson, "Today's View in Maternal and Fetal Medicine," *Patient Care*, 1983, as cited in Hubbard, *The Politics of Women's Biology*, 176.

36. Ibid.

37. Rayna Rapp, "Real Time Is Prime Time: The Role of the Sonogram in the Age of Mechanical Reproduction," in *Cyborgs and Citadels: Anthropological Interventions into Techno-Medicine*, ed. G. Downey, J. Dunit, and Sharon Traweek (Seattle: University of Washington Press, forthcoming).

38. Carol A. Stabile offers an incisive reading of *Life*'s 1965 cover photo "Drama of Life Before Birth" and its 1990 counterpart, "The First Days of Creation," in "Shooting the Mother: Fetal Photography and the Politics of Disappearance," *camera obscura* 28 (1992): 178–205.

39. M. Johnson and B. Everitt, *Essential Reproduction* (Oxford: Blackwell Scientific Publications, 1988), 265, cited in Franklin, "Fetal Fascinations," 193.

40. Horatio R. Storer and Franklin Fiske Heard, *Criminal Abortion: Its Nature, Its Evidence, and Its Law* (Boston: Little, Brown, 1868), 10–11, cited in Reva Siegel, "Reasoning from the Body: A Historical Perspective on Abortion Regulation and Questions of Equal Protection," *Stanford Law Review* 44 (1992): 326.

41. Patrick Steptoe, cited in Sarah Franklin, "Essentialism, Which Essentialism? Some Implications of Reproductive and Genetic Techno-Science," *Journal of Homosexuality* 24, nos. 3–4 (1993): 31.

42. Patrick Steptoe, observation made at the Women, Reproduction, and Technology

Conference, History Workshop Centre, Oxford, February 14–15, 1987, cited in Michelle Stanworth, "The Deconstruction of Motherhood," in *Reproductive Technologies: Gender, Motherhood, and Medicine*, ed. Michelle Stanworth (Minneapolis: University of Minnesota Press, 1987), 15.

43. The literature that pertains here is far too rich to exhaust in a single note. To get a sense of the diverse framings of this point, see, for example, Donna Haraway, "The Promise of Monsters: A Regenerative Politics for Inappropriate/d Others," in *Cultural Studies*, ed. Lawrence Grossberg, Cary Nelson, and Paula A. Treichler (New York: Routledge, 1992); Donna Hawaray, *Simians, Cyborgs, and Women: The Reinvention of Nature* (New York: Routledge, 1991), especially chap. 9; Evelyn Fox Keller, *Secrets of Life, Secrets of Death: Essays on Language, Gender and Science* (New York: Routledge, 1992); Michael Ryan and Avery Gordon, eds., *Body Politics: Disease, Desire, and the Family* (Boulder, Colo.: Westview, 1994); Mary Jacobus, Evelyn Fox Keller, and Sally Shuttleworth, eds., *Body/Politics: Women and the Discourses of Science* (New York: Routledge, 1990); Chris Hables Gray, ed., with Heidi J. Figueroa-Sarriera and Steven Mentor, *The Cyborg Handbook* (New York: Routledge, 1995).

2 / Containing Women: Reproductive Discourse(s) in the 1980s

1. Thomas G. Keane, "Brain-Dead Mother Has Her Baby," *San Francisco Chronicle*, July 31, 1986.

2. "Out of Death, a New Life Comes," *Newsweek*, April 1, 1983, 65.

3. "Giving Life after Death: Two Stories," *Newsweek*, August 11, 1986, 48.

4. Ibid. Following the extraction of a viable fetus from the body of a brain-dead woman, Dr. Russell K. Laros Jr. had this to say: "The experience left me with real confidence that this can be done without any great difficulties. . . . In the future, I'll suggest to family members that the option is there." From *OB/GYN News*, June 1, 1983, quoted in Gena Corea, *The Mother Machine: Reproductive Technologies from Artificial Insemination to Artificial Wombs* (New York: Harper & Row, 1985), 281.

5. "Orphan Embryos Saved," *San Francisco Chronicle*, October 24, 1984.

6. Peter Singer and Deane Wells, *Making Babies: The New Science and Ethics of Conception* (New York: Charles Scribner's Sons, 1985), 87.

7. Ibid.

8. On this understanding—from the obvious to the obtuse—there exists a rich and ever-expanding feminist literature.

9. Rosalind Petchesky, "Abortion, the Church and the State," unpublished manuscript (1985), 15; Zillah Eisenstein, "The Sexual Politics of the New Right: The 'Crisis of Liberalism' for the 1980s," *Signs* 7 (1982): 567–88.

10. Rosalind Petchesky, "Antiabortion, Antifeminism, and the Rise of the New Right," *Feminist Studies* 2 (1981): 206–46.

11. *Roe v. Wade*, 410 U.S. 113 (1973), 159.

12. Gary Jacobsohn, *The Supreme Court and the Decline of Constitutional Aspiration* (Totowa, N.J.: Rowman & Littlefield, 1986), 131.

13. *Roe v. Wade*, 157–59, 161–62.

14. Daniel Wikler, "Abortion, Privacy and Personhood: From Roe v. Wade to the Human Life Statute," in *Abortion: Moral and Legal Perspectives*, ed. Jay L. Garfield and Patricia Hennesey (Amherst: University of Massachusetts Press, 1984), 252.

15. Resolution of the National Academy of Science, April 28, 1981, cited in Laurence Tribe, "Prepared Statement before the United States Senate on the Human Life Bill," in

Abortion, Medicine and the Law, ed. J. Douglas Butler and David F. Walbert (New York: Facts on File, 1986), appendix 2, n. 5, 493.

16. Ibid., 481.

17. "For where-ever any two Men are, who have no standing Rule, and common Judge to Appeal to on Earth for the determination of Controversies of Right betwixt them, they are in the State of Nature, and under all the inconveniences of it." John Locke, *Two Treatises of Government*, ed. Peter Laslett (New York: New American Library, 1963), 2:91. "It may be perceived what manner of life there would be, where there were no common power to fear. . . . In such a condition, there is no place for industry . . . no culture of the earth; no navigation . . . no commodious building . . . no account of time; no arts; no letters; no society; and which is worst of all, continual fear and danger of violent death; and the life of man, solitary, poor, nasty, brutish, and short." Thomas Hobbes, *Leviathan*, ed. Michael Oakeshott (New York: Collier, 1974), 101, 100.

18. A letter to the editor that appeared in the progressive paper *In These Times,* by a woman representing herself as "pro-choice for many years" but now "pro-life," gives an account of these hearings that, although riddled with inaccuracies, is clear testimony to their success in giving the impression that the issue of fetal personhood has indeed been "solved" and in objectively defensible terms. The author writes: "In congressional hearings not long after Roe v. Wade, the question of when the exact moment human life begins was explored by top physicians and biologists from around the U.S. Everyone who testified, whether pro-life or pro-choice, said the same thing—human life begins at the moment of conception. Given this statement, it is inconceivable that any group that promulgates itself as one that upholds the rights of all against exploiters could possibly support elective abortions." *In These Times* 13, no. 16 (1989): 15.

19. Janet Gallagher, "Fetal Personhood and Women's Policy," in *Women, Biology, and Public Policy,* ed. Virginia Sapiro (Beverly Hills: Sage, 1985).

20. Rosalind Petchesky, "Fetal Images: The Power of Visual Culture in the Politics of Reproduction," in *Reproductive Technologies: Gender, Motherhood, and Medicine,* ed. Michelle Stanworth (Minneapolis: University of Minnesota Press, 1987), 29.

21. Ibid., 62.

22. Joseph C. Fletcher and Mark I. Evans, "Maternal Bonding in Early Fetal Ultrasound Examinations," *New England Journal of Medicine* 308 (1983): 392–93.

23. Ibid., 392. Caroline Whitbeck tells of a "Boston obstetrician who subjects her patients to ultrasound imaging every month of pregnancy for the purpose of 'helping the woman bond to her baby.'" "Fetal Imaging and Fetal Monitoring: Finding the Ethical Issues," in *Embryos, Ethics, and Women's Rights,* ed. Elaine Hoffman Barauch, Amadeo F. D'Adamo Jr, and Joni Seagar (New York: Harrington Park, 1988), 56.

24. Petchesky, "Fetal Images," 59.

25. Ibid.

26. These technical advances stoke the quite distorted popular impression that fetuses now capable of survival can be (and are being) aborted, legally. Able-baby survival of twenty-four-week-old fetuses is still quite rare—indeed, considerably less than 50 percent. Also important to keep in mind is that less than .01 percent of all abortions actually occur between the twenty-fourth and twenty-sixth weeks of pregnancy.

27. Gallagher, "Fetal Personhood," 92.

28. Bernard Nathanson, *The Abortion Papers: Inside the Abortion Mentality* (New York: Frederick Fell, 1983), 16–17. Indeed, so convinced was Nathanson that the various new techniques of fetal therapy and repair "revealed" the personhood of the fetus, he quit his New York City-based abortion practice and joined the crusade to recriminal-

ize the procedure. "What persuaded me to change my mind [regarding the life status of the fetus] was the marvelous new technology which has served to define beyond reasonable challenge the nature of interuterine life, the inarguably and specifically human quality of that life. Where is the scientific evidence, where are the new developments which would serve to convince us of the contrary view, that what is in the uterus from the beginning of pregnancy is less human today than that which we perceived in 1965. We had no ultrasound in those years, no fetal heart monitoring, no fetoscopy, no invitro fertilization. Science marches inexorably towards a deeper understanding of the uniquely human qualities of the fetus."

29. Michael R. Harrison, "Unborn: Historical Perspectives of the Fetus as Patient," *Pharos* (Winter 1982): 19–24, quoted in Ruth Hubbard, "Personal Courage is Not Enough: Some Hazards of Childbearing in the 1980s," in *Test-Tube Women*, ed. Rita Arditti, Renate Duelli Klein, and Shelly Minden (Boston: Pandora, 1984), 348–49.

30. Frederic Frigolleto, quoted in Lucy H. Labson, "Today's View in Maternal and Fetal Medicine," *Patient Care,* 1983, 105, as quoted in Hubbard, "Personal Courage Is Not Enough," 349.

31. Hubbard, "Personal Courage Is Not Enough," 349.

32. Notwithstanding the slippage in public discourse between "patienthood" and "personhood," it seems worth noting here that *patienthood* is fundamentally a relational term, whereas *personhood* is not, at least not as the word is conventionally used and understood.

33. *Nightline,* April 7, 1989.

34. The point is not that technologies facilitate only reactionary conclusions and uses, but that the context/relations, the "who," determines in toto what is seen; clearly, with these same technologies we could see and conclude other things.

35. Jacques Le Goff, "Head or Heart? The Political Use of Body Metaphors in the Middle Ages," in *Fragments for a History of the Human Body: Part Three,* ed. Michael Feher with Romina Naddaff and Nadia Tazi (Cambridge, Mass.: Zone, 1988), 13–26.

36. On the effects of liberalized abortion, see, for example, Dan Baker, *Beyond Choice: The Abortion Story No One Is Telling* (Portland, Ore.: Multnomah, 1985); Ann Saltenberger, *Every Woman Has a Right to Know the Dangers of Legal Abortion* (Glassboro, N.J.: Air-Plus Enterprises, 1983), especially chaps. 6–8.

37. Marvin Kohl, *The Morality of Killing: Sanctity of Life, Abortion, and Euthanasia* (New York: Humanities Press, 1974), cited in Barbara Hayler, "Review Essay: Abortion," *Signs* 4 (1979): 322–33.

38. In Reagan's own words, as reported in Jay Cocks, "How Long Till Equality?" *Time,* July 12, 1982, 23: "Part of the reason for the high unemployment 'is not so much recession as it is the great increase in people going into the job market, and ladies, I'm not picking on anyone, but [it is] because of the increase in women who are working today and two-worker families.'"

39. Phyllis Schlafly, *The Power of the Positive Woman* (New York: Jove, 1977), 78, 212.

40. Interview with prolife activist in Kristen Luker, *Abortion and the Politics of Motherhood* (Berkeley: University of California Press, 1984), 159–60.

41. Gina Kolata, "Operating on the Unborn," *New York Times Magazine,* May 14, 1989, 35.

42. Rex B. Wintgerter, "Fetal Protection Becomes Assault on Motherhood," *In These Times,* June 10–23, 1987; Nan Hunter, "Feticide: Cases and Legislation," memorandum to the ACLU, Reproductive Freedom Project (May 5, 1986).

43. Nan Hunter, "State Legislation Concerning 'Feticide' and 'Wrongful Birth/

Wrongful Life,'" memorandum to ACLU Affiliates, Reproductive Freedom Project (April 15, 1983).

44. Fetal protection statutes clearly affect all women of childbearing age, but they operate with additional cruelty against women who lack class and/or race privilege. The very conditions of these women's lives indict them: poverty, lack of access to adequate health and quality medical care, and often toxic environmental living and working conditions constitute what the courts would call "negligent fetal injuries." For a fuller discussion of fetal protection statutes, see Cynthia R. Daniels, *At Women's Expense: State Power and the Politics of Fetal Rights* (Cambridge: Harvard University Press, 1993); Sally J. Kenny, *For Whose Protection? Reproductive Hazards and Exclusionary Policies in the United States and Britain* (Ann Arbor: University of Michigan Press, 1992).

45. George J. Annas, "Pregnant Women as Fetal Containers," *Hastings Center Report* 16, no. 6 (1986): 14; Gallagher, "Fetal Personhood," 104–5.

46. Gallagher, "Fetal Personhood," 106. See also Dawn E. Johnsen, "The Creation of Fetal Rights: Conflicts with Women's Constitutional Rights to Liberty, Privacy, and Equal Protection," *Yale Law Journal* 95 (1986): 599–625.

47. Zillah Eisenstein appears to make a similar point and to develop similar themes in *The Female Body and the Law* (Berkeley: University of California Press, 1988). See also Reva Siegel, "Reasoning from the Body: A Historical Perspective on Abortion Regulation and Questions of Equal Protection," *Stanford Law Review* 44 (1992): 261–381.

48. Although pregnant women can be forced to abstain from "unhealthy" behavior, undergo blood transfusions, or have major surgery for the good of the fetus, courts would never coerce an adult male (or female) to undergo, for example, a bone marrow transplant for the good of a son or daughter, mother, cousin, brother, friend, even if he (or she) happens to be the only compatible donor. In adjudicating such a situation, a Pittsburgh judge had this to say: "Morally, this decision rests with the defendant and, in the view of the Court, the refusal of the defendant is morally indefensible. [But] to *compel* the Defendant to submit to an intrusion of his body would change every concept and principle upon which our society is founded. To do so would defeat the sanctity of the individual and would impose a rule which would know no limits and one could not imagine where the line would be drawn." *McFall v. Schimp*, cited in Gallagher, "Fetal Personhood," 106.

49. The image here is similar in mood to the one Euripides creates in *The Bacchae* (Chicago: University of Chicago Press, 1958), lines 1200–1308: Agave's moment of recognition and horror when she sees clearly that the "lion" she has hunted and savagely (not to mention ecstatically) dismembered under the spell of Dionysus is in fact her own son.

50. Maggie Garb, "Abortion Foes Give Birth to a 'Syndrome,'" *In These Times*, February 22–March 1, 1989, 3; Nada L. Stotland, "Commentary: The Myth of the Abortion Trauma Syndrome," *Journal of the American Medical Association* 269 (1992): 2078–79.

51. Women Exploited by Abortion, "Before You Make the Decision," pamphlet (n.d.).

52. Jill Eisen, "Drawing the Line: Reproductive Technologies," transcript of CBC *Ideas*, March 17 and 24, 1986, 1, cited in Christine Overall, *Ethics and Human Reproduction: A Feminist Analysis* (Boston: Allen & Unwin, 1987), 142.

53. See, for example, Peter Roberts, "The Brennen Story: A Small Miracle of Creation," in *Test-Tube Babies*, ed. Peter Singer and William Walters (Melbourne: Oxford University Press, 1982), especially 13–16; Isabel Bainbridge, "With Child in Mind: The Experience of a Potential IVF Mother," also in *Test-Tube Babies*, especially 120–22.

54. "The Saddest Epidemic," *Time*, September 10, 1984, 50.

55. Patrick Steptoe, observation made at the Women, Reproduction, and Technology Conference, History Workshop Centre, Oxford, February 14–15, 1987, cited in Michelle Stanworth, "Reproduction and the Deconstruction of Motherhood," in *Reproductive Technologies: Gender, Motherhood, and Medicine*, ed. Michelle Stanworth (Minneapolis: University of Minnesota Press, 1987), 15.

56. This statistic is from Ann Snitow, "The Paradox of Birth Technology: Exploring the Good, the Bad and the Scary," *Ms.*, December 1986, 48.

57. *Life*, June 1987.

58. When particular groups of women (and men) are seen as "breeders," their infertility comes to be regarded as a "solution" rather than a problem.

59. Susan E. Davies, ed., *Women under Attack: Victories, Backlash and the Fight for Reproductive Freedom*, Pamphlet 7, Committee for Abortion Rights and Against Sterilization Abuse (Boston: South End, 1988), 31.

60. Carl Wood and Ann Westmore, *Test-Tube Conception* (Englewood Cliffs, N.J.: Prentice Hall, 1983), 96.

61. "Visions of Tomorrow," *Life*, February 1989, 54–55.

62. "Giving Life after Death."

63. "Visions of Tomorrow," 55.

64. Robert Hanley, "Father of Baby M Granted Custody: Contract Upheld," *New York Times*, April 1, 1987, A1.

65. About the preferability of ectogenesis or extracorporeal reproduction to surrogacy, Singer and Wells themselves continue: "If, for instance, early experience with surrogacy showed that surrogate *mothers* could not be relied upon to give up *to their genetic parents* the children they had carried, ectogenesis might be thought better than a battle over custody. Evidence that surrogate mothers frequently smoked or took alcohol or drugs that caused harm to the *baby* might be another reason for preferring the strictly controlled artificial environment." *Making Babies*, 119, emphasis added.

66. Mary Meehan, "Abortion: The Left Has Betrayed the Sanctity of Life," *The Progressive*, September 1980, cited in Nat Hentoff, "How Can the Left Be Against Life?" *Village Voice*, July 18, 1985, 17.

67. Robert Smothers, "Embryos in a Divorce Case: Joint Property or Offspring?" *New York Times*, April 22, 1989, A1.

68. Ibid.

69. "Rescue Urged for Frozen Embryos," *San Francisco Chronicle*, August 11, 1989. The conceptual confusion in the analogy is that this woman simultaneously becomes Eichman and the Allied troops. Moreover, to fulfill her "rescue mission" all seven "preborn children" must be implanted and brought to term—an undertaking fundamentally at odds with the very rationale of multiple egg harvesting for achieving an IVF pregnancy.

70. Ibid.

3 / Fetal Exposures: Abortion Politics and the Optics of Allusion

1. Sarah Franklin, "Fetal Fascinations: New Dimensions to the Medical-Scientific Construction of Fetal Personhood," in *Off-Centre: Feminism and Cultural Studies*, ed. Sarah Franklin, Celia Lury, and Jackie Stacey (New York: HarperCollins, 1991), 195.

2. *The Miracle of Life*, Swedish television production in association with WGBH Educational Foundation, Boston; aired on the PBS program *Nova* in 1986.

3. The phrase is Sarah Franklin's; see "Fetal Fascinations," 195.

4. For an engaging analysis of the complex rhetorical efforts entailed in generating a meaningful fetal image, see Celeste Michelle Condit, *Decoding Abortion Rhetoric: Communicating Social Change* (Chicago: University of Illinois Press, 1990), 79–92. Additional and provocative studies include those by Rosalind Petchesky, "Fetal Images: The Power of Visual Culture in the Politics of Reproduction," in *Reproductive Technologies: Gender, Motherhood, and Medicine*, ed. Michelle Stanworth (Minneapolis: University of Minnesota Press, 1987), 57–80; Franklin, "Fetal Fascinations," 190–205; Janelle S. Taylor, "The Public Fetus and the Family Car: From Abortion Politics to a Volvo Advertisement," *Public Culture* 4, no. 2 (1992): 67–80.

5. *S'Aline's Solution* was one of six videos shown in December 1991 at the University of California, San Diego, under the auspices of a program titled "The Bad Body." Curated by video artist Julie Zando and sponsored by the university's Visual Arts Department, the program featured the work of avant-garde video makers on a variety of topics within the field of body politics.

6. On the links among ultrasound imaging, maternal bonding, and abortion, see Joseph C. Fletcher and Mark I. Evans, "Maternal Bonding in Early Fetal Ultrasound Examinations," *New England Journal of Medicine* 308 (1983): 392–93. I do not mean to imply in this discussion that the experience of loss some women experience following aborted pregnancies is imagined or contrived. Rather, my point is that the *public discourse of loss* both simplifies and exploits the variety of women's experiences and struggles with respect to abortion—the often ambivalent and complicated feelings that attend any "serious" act—to reinscribe and enforce a narrow, ideologically biologistic understanding of gender and motherhood.

7. Or so we are led to believe. It is worth mentioning, if only in passing, that what *Nova* presents and we accept as a fantastic voyage through the exotic interiors of the natural body might be just that—"fantastic" as in phantasmagoric. Here, as with *S'Aline's Solution*, we take on faith the truth of the image and do not question where we are or what we are seeing.

8. Faye D. Ginsburg, "The 'Word-Made-Flesh,'" in *Uncertain Terms: Negotiating Gender in American Culture*, ed. Faye D. Ginsburg and Anna Lowenhaupt Tsing (Boston: Beacon, 1990), 68–69.

9. For especially provocative discussions of these and related issues, see Donna Haraway, "Situated Knowledges," in *Simians, Cyborgs, and Women: The Reinvention of Nature* (New York: Routledge, 1991), 183–201; and Haraway's "The Promise of Monsters: A Regenerative Politics for Inappropriate/d Others," in *Cultural Studies*, ed. Lawrence Grossberg, Cary Nelson, and Paula A. Treichler (New York: Routledge, 1992), 295–337.

10. This point is drawn from and developed further by Rayna Rapp in "Constructing Amniocentesis: Maternal and Medical Discourses," in *Uncertain Terms: Negotiating Gender in American Culture*, ed. Faye D. Ginsberg and Anna Lowenhaupt Tsing (Boston: Beacon, 1990), 41.

11. For these statistics, see *Abortion: For Survival*, a video produced by the Fund for the Feminist Majority, 1989.

12. For a more detailed analysis of the forces and issues at play in the legalization of abortion, see Rosalind Petchesky, *Abortion and Woman's Choice: The State, Sexuality, and Reproductive Freedom* (New York: Longman, 1984), particularly 101–33.

13. As Sarah Franklin explains, "The very term 'individual,' meaning *one who cannot be divided*, can only mean the male, as it is precisely the process of one individual becoming two which occurs through a woman's pregnancy. Pregnancy is precisely about

one body becoming two bodies, two bodies becoming one, the exact antithesis of individuality. This is, claims Donna Haraway, 'why women have had so much trouble counting as individuals in modern western discourses. Their personal, bounded individuality is compromised by their bodies' troubling talent for making other bodies, whose individuality can take precedence over their own.'" "Fetal Fascinations," 203. Franklin's quote from Haraway is found in Donna Haraway, "The Biopolitics of Postmodern Bodies: Determinations of Self in Immune System Discourse," *differences* 1, no. 1 (1988): 39.

14. The recent indiscriminate display at prolife rallies of "actual" fetal corpses alongside pictures of fetuses, both serene and gruesome, reflects and reinforces precisely such a misreading. Also contributing to this kind of misreading is a new series of commercials being aired on national television that portray children of all ages and races—potential abortees—frolicking about in joyful play. Each commercial ends with the statement, "Life, what a beautiful choice." One particularly striking commercial in this series depicts a woman singing "Amazing Grace" in a choir. The voice-over, presumably the woman herself, explains that she was an aborted fetus who nevertheless survived the attempt on her life. Speaking as a postnatal fetus on behalf of her prenatal counterparts, she cautions viewers about making the same mistake that was made with respect to her.

15. The argument goes something like this: since the Supreme Court handed down its ruling in *Roe v. Wade,* knowledge about the nature of fetal life as well as technological interventions to support that life have advanced dramatically, thus forcing the already complicated range of moral questions entailed in the practice of choice to be fundamentally refigured. That we increasingly treat the fetus as person/patient is generally thought to have something to do with these advances revealing its "true" or "essential" nature as such. As I have been both suggesting and implying throughout this essay, however, fetal personhood is not a "property" that can or will be "discovered" with greater scientific knowledge or increased technological capabilities, but is produced in and through the very practices that claim merely to "reveal" it.

16. The phrase is Sarah Franklin's; see "Fetal Fascinations," 196.

4 / Reproducing Public Meanings: In the Matter of Baby M

1. Letter to the editor, *New York Times*, February 18, 1988, A2.

2. "Matter of Baby M," Superior Court of New Jersey, Bergen County (March 31, 1987), 58–62.

3. Quoted in Otto Friedrich, "A Legal, Moral, and Social Nightmare: Society Seeks to Define the Problems of the Birth Revolution," *Time*, September 10, 1984, 55. For an interesting discussion of the ways in which "questions posed by reproductive technologies [and surrogacy in particular] challenge the most basic tenets of family law," see Andrea E. Stumpf, "Redefining Mother: A Legal Matrix for New Reproductive Technologies," *Yale Law Journal* 96 (1986): 187–208.

4. Quoted in Friedrich, "A Legal, Moral, and Social Nightmare," 54.

5. "Matter of Baby M," 73, 71.

6. "Baby M," Supreme Court of New Jersey, 537 A.2D 1227, *1234.

7. Ibid., *1240.

8. Ibid., *1246.

9. Ibid., *1248.

10. Ibid., *1238.

11. James Boyd White, *Justice as Translation: An Essay in Cultural and Legal Criticism* (Chicago: University of Chicago Press, 1990), 135.

12. I am not suggesting that the world Sorkow's ruling produces is one in which there are literally no women; rather, it is a world in which women do not count in any substantive sense. Within the logic of paternity, women function as the nurture/nature context for life; they are but soil for the seed. For a provocative and engaging discussion of these issues, see Carol Delaney, "The Meaning of Paternity and the Virgin Birth Debate," *Man* 21 (1986): 494–513. On the operation of juridical discourse, see Jane M. Gaines, *Contested Culture: The Image, the Voice, and the Law* (Chapel Hill: University of North Carolina Press, 1991), 11–18.

13. Michel Foucault, *History of Sexuality,* vol. 1 (New York: Vintage, 1980), 86. "We must make allowance for the complex and unstable process whereby discourse can be both an instrument and an effect of power, but also a hindrance, stumbling-block, a point of resistance and a starting point for an opposing strategy. Discourse transmits and produces power; it reinforces it, but also undermines and exposes it, renders it fragile and makes it possible to thwart it" (101).

14. White, *Justice as Translation,* 101; see also James Boyd White, "Constituting a Culture of Argument: The Possibilities of American Law," in *When Words Lose Their Meaning: Constitutions and Reconstitutions of Language, Character, and Community* (Chicago: University of Chicago Press, 1984), 231–74; Mary Ann Glendon, *Abortion and Divorce in Western Law* (Cambridge: Harvard University Press, 1987), especially chap. 1.

15. This is now fairly common understanding among feminists and critical legal theorists even if it is also contested within the broader community of legal scholarship. See, for example, Carol Smart, *Feminism and the Power of Law* (New York: Routledge, 1989); Zillah Eisenstein, *The Female Body and the Law* (Berkeley: University of California Press, 1988), especially chap. 2; Patricia J. Williams, *The Alchemy of Race and Rights* (Cambridge: Harvard University Press, 1991).

16. Mary Beth Whitehead with Loretta Schwartz-Nobel, *A Mother's Story* (New York: St. Martin's, 1989), 7.

17. "Matter of Baby M," 28.

18. In traditional surrogacy, a married, heterosexual couple hires a "surrogate" who is then artificially inseminated with the male's sperm, gestates the embryo/fetus, to which she is genetically related, and surrenders it upon birth. In gestational surrogacy, a surrogate is hired to gestate the embryo of a married, heterosexual couple that has been fertilized in vitro and to which she bears no genetic relationship.

19. Kim Lane Scheppele, "Facing Facts in Legal Interpretation," *Representations* 30 (1990). 60.

20. "Matter of Baby M," 13–15.

21. Ibid., 13, 14.

22. Ibid., 16.

23. For a recent pessimistic reading of fertility treatments, see Sharon Begley, "Infertility: Has the Hype Outweighed the Hope?" *Newsweek*, September 4, 1995, 38–45. The sad irony here is that *Newsweek*—among other popular newsmagazines—in its utter pronatal infatuation with new reproductive innovations, contributed throughout the 1980s to what it now derisively characterizes as "the baby myth."

24. These causes of infertility are cited in Ann Snitow, "The Paradox of Birth Technology: Exploring the Good, the Bad, and the Scary," *Ms.*, December 1986, 48.

25. "Matter of Baby M," 15.

26. Ibid., 71, 108. Elsewhere in the ruling, Judge Sorkow states, "Use of laws not intended for their intended purpose creates forced and confusing results" (74).

27. Ibid., 73, 71.

28. For ruminations on "paternity," see Thomas W. Laqueur, "The Facts of Fatherhood," in *Conflicts in Feminism*, ed. Marianne Hirsch and Evelyn Fox Keller (New York: Routledge, 1990), 205–21.

29. Jean-Pierre Vernant, *Myth and Thought among the Greeks* (London: Routledge, 1983), 134. See also Pierre Videl-Naquet, "Aeschylus, the Past, and the Present," in *Myth and Tragedy in Ancient Greece*, ed. Jean-Pierre Vernant and Pierre Videl-Naquet (New York: Zone, 1988), 266; Froma Zeitlin, "The Dynamics of Misogyny: Myth and Mythmaking in the *Oresteia*," *Arethusa* 11 (1978): 149–77.

30. Vernant, *Myth and Thought*, 134.

31. Aeschylus, *Oresteia*, trans. Richard Lattimore (Chicago: University of Chicago Press, 1953), ll. 658–61.

32. Ibid., ll. 662–66.

33. G. E. R. Lloyd, ed., *Hippocratic Writings*, trans. J. Chadwick and W. N. Mann (New York: Penguin, 1978), 317–20. See also Aristotle, *Generation of Animals*, trans. A. L. Peck (Cambridge: Harvard University Press, 1979), 103–13; Plato, *Timaeus*, trans. Desmond Lee (New York: Penguin, 1977), 122–24. Zeitlin elaborates, "The major component of semen is *pneuma*, a foamlike airy substance which contains the seed of the divine. Originating in the brain, semen is responsible for endowing offspring with the essential human capacity for reason, for logos. Seed of generation, of intellectual ability, and of the divine element in the human species, semen confirms the innate superiority of male over female." "The Dynamics of Misogyny," 169.

34. Aeschylus, *Oresteia*, ll. 736–40.

35. "When Melissa was born on March 27, 1986, there was not attendant to the circumstance of her birth the family gatherings, the family celebrations or the family worship services that usually accompany such a happy family event. . . . In reality, the fact of family was undefined of non-existant [sic]. The mother and father are known but they are not family. The interposition of their spouses will not serve to create family without further court intervention." "Matter of Baby M," 111.

36. Perhaps more to the point here is Judge Sorkow's argument that the terms of the surrogacy contract are fixed with conception. Sperm seals the deal: "This court holds . . . that in New Jersey, although the surrogacy contract is signed, the surrogate may nevertheless renounce and terminate the contract until the time of conception. . . . once conception has occurred the parties are fixed, the terms of the contract are firm and performance will be anticipated with the joy that only a newborn can bring." "Matter of Baby M," 75.

37. Ibid., 91.

38. Janet L. Dolgin, "Status and Contract in Surrogate Motherhood: An Illumination of the Surrogacy Debate," *Buffalo Law Review* 38 (1990): 538–39.

39. "Matter of Baby M," 45–46. Janice Doane and Devon Hodges offer a somewhat more thorough discussion of the family form fashioned by Sorkow in "Risky Business: Familial Ideology and the Case of Baby M," *differences* 1, no. 1 (1989): 67–81.

40. "Matter of Baby M," 46.

41. "Baby M," *1248.

42. Ibid., *1249.

43. I am thinking in particular of the arguments proffered by John Stuart Mill in *The Subjection of Women*, ed. Sue Mansfield (Arlington Heights, Ill.: Harlan Davidson, 1980); Mary Wollstonecraft, *A Vindication of the Rights of Women*, ed. Carol H. Pos-

ton (New York: W. W. Norton, 1975); and Jean-Jacques Rousseau, *Emile; or, On Education*, trans. Allan Bloom (New York: Basic Books, 1979). For a general discussion of gender as text and subtext in liberal discourse, see Carole Pateman, *The Disorder of Women: Democracy, Feminism, and Political Theory* (Stanford, Calif.: Stanford University Press, 1989); Carole Pateman, *The Sexual Contract* (Stanford, Calif.: Stanford University Press, 1988); and Jane Rendall, "Virtue and Commerce: Women in the Making of Adam Smith's Political Economy," in *Women in Western Political Philosophy*, ed. Ellen Kennedy and Susan Mendus (New York: St. Martin's, 1987), 44–77.

44. On this division and the ways in which it serves as an elaborate institutional mechanism to both constitute and sustain male prerogative and paternal right, see Pateman, *The Disorder of Women*, especially chaps. 1, 6, 8; Pateman, *The Sexual Contract*; Nancy Fraser, "What's Critical about Critical Theory? The Case of Habermass and Gender," in *Unruly Practices: Power, Discourse, and Gender in Contemporary Social Theory* (Minneapolis: University of Minnesota Press, 1989), especially 127–37; Mary O'Brien, *The Politics of Reproduction* (London: Routledge, 1981); Genevieve Lloyd, *The Man of Reason: "Male" and "Female" in Western Philosophy* (Minneapolis: University of Minnesota Press, 1984); Anne Phillips, *Engendering Democracy* (Cambridge: Polity, 1991).

45. Fraser, "What's Critical about Critical Theory?" 122.

46. Teresa de Lauretis, "The Technology of Gender," in *Technologies of Gender* (Bloomington: Indiana University Press, 1987), 3.

47. "Baby M," *1259.

48. Dolgin, "Status and Contract," 540.

49. Ibid., 537.

50. "Baby M," *1258, *1260.

51. Lest it seem this argument is overly exercised with respect to the the court's findings, see Katharine T. Bartlett, "Re-expressing Parenthood," *Yale Law Journal* 98 (1988): "The best interest of the child is a highly contingent social construction. Although we often pretend otherwise, it seems clear that our judgements about what is best for children are as much the result of political and social judgements about what kind of society we prefer as they are conclusions based upon neutral or scientific data about what is 'best' for children. The resolution of conflicts over children ultimately is less a matter of objective fact-finding than it is a matter of deciding what kind of children and families—what kind of relationships—we want to have" (295).

52. Jana Sawicki, *Disciplining Foucault: Feminism, Power, and the Body* (New York: Routledge, 1991), 88.

5 / Breached Birth: Anna Johnson and the Reproduction of Raced Bodies

1. Quoted in Catherine Gewertz, "Surrogate Mother Sues to Keep Couple's Child," *Los Angeles Times*, August 14, 1990, A1.

2. Ibid., A22.

3. Although Johnson may have been approached by various talk shows, in point of fact, she appeared only on *Donahue* in order to counter what she took to be widespread media misrepresentations of her claims. Although Johnson apparently received payment for her appearance—forty-six hundred dollars, or precisely the amount she required to repay Social Services—she testified that she knew nothing of this payment

and did not personally receive it. Although this seems, on the surface, to be somewhat far-fetched, it is entirely possible that any fee Johnson received for her appearance was negotiated by and channeled through her lawyers. Contrary to public perceptions, talk-show guests rarely receive compensation for their participation beyond airfare and hotel accommodations.

4. Catherine Gewertz, "Surrogate Mother in Custody Fight Accused of Welfare Fraud," *Los Angeles Times,* August 16, 1990, A10.

5. Wahneema Lubiano, "Black Ladies, Welfare Queens, and State Minstrels: Ideological War by Narrative Means," in *Race-ing Justice, En-gendering Power: Essays on Anita Hill, Clarence Thomas, and the Construction of Social Reality,* ed. Toni Morrison (New York: Pantheon, 1992), 338–39.

6. See Kobena Mercer, *Welcome to the Jungle: New Positions in Black Cultural Studies* (New York: Routledge, 1994), especially chap. 5.

7. Michael de Courcey Hinds, "Addiction to Crack Can Kill Parental Instinct," *New York Times,* March 17, 1990, A1.

8. On illegitimate birthrates, see Susan Faludi, *Backlash: The Undeclared War against American Women* (New York: Anchor, 1991), 34.

9. Lubiano, "Black Ladies," 331.

10. The significant passage of the act upon which Johnson's lawyers depended provides that the relationship "between a child and the natural mother may be established by proof of her having given birth to the child."

11. "In the committee's view, the genetic link between the commissioning parent(s) and the resulting infant, while important is less weighty than the link between the surrogate mother and fetus or infant that is created through gestation at birth. Thus, in the analysis and recommendations that follow, no distinction will be drawn between the usual pattern of surrogate parenting and surrogate gestational motherhood." "Ethical Issues in Surrogate Motherhood," trial exhibit, *Johnson v. Calvert,* Office of the Supreme Court, California (1990), 2.

12. Gina Kolata, "Menopause Is Found No Bar to Pregnancy," *New York Times,* October 25, 1990, A1.

13. "That the egg is not their own is a detail; what counts is that they are able to have a profound and transforming life experience, to bond prenatally with their baby, and reproduce the genes of their husband." Katha Pollitt, "When Is a Mother Not a Mother?" *The Nation,* December 31, 1990, 844.

14. Interview with prolife activist in Kristen Luker, *Abortion and the Politics of Motherhood* (Berkeley: University of California Press, 1984), 159–60.

15. Joseph C. Fletcher and Mark I. Evans, "Maternal Bonding in Early Fetal Ultrasound Examinations," *New England Journal of Medicine* 308 (1983): 392.

16. For a fuller discussion, see Rosalind Petchesky, "Fetal Images: The Power of Visual Culture in the Politics of Reproduction," in *Reproductive Technologies: Gender, Motherhood, and Medicine,* ed. Michelle Stanworth (Minneapolis: University of Minnesota Press, 1987), 59.

17. Carol Whitbeck, "Fetal Imaging and Fetal Monitoring: Finding the Ethical Issues," in *Embryos, Ethics, and Women's Rights,* ed. Elaine Hoffman Baruch, Amadeo F. D'Adamo Jr., and Joni Seager (New York: Harrington Park, 1988), 56.

18. "Three natural parents is not in the best interest of the child. . . . I think it invites emotional and financial extortion situations." Trial transcript, *Johnson v. Calvert,* 1488.

19. Ibid., 1489–90.

20. Ibid., 1489.

21. Ibid., 1483–84.

22. Janet L. Dolgin, "Family Law and the Facts of Family," unpublished manuscript (1992), 34. A version of this paper was published as "Just a Gene: Judicial Assumptions about Parenthood," *UCLA Law Review* 40 (1993): 637–94.

23. Trial transcript, *Johnson v. Calvert*, 1490.

24. Ibid., 1487, 918–20.

25. "Who we are and what we are and identity problems particularly with young children and teenagers are extremely important. We know that there is a combination of genetic factors. We know more and more about traits now, how you walk, talk, and everything else, all sorts of things that develop out of your genes, how long you're going to live, all things being equal, when your immune system is going to break down, what diseases you may be susceptible to. They have upped the intelligence ratio to 70 percent now. Then there is environment. Over the years the experts flow back and forth between how much is genetics and how much is environment after you're born. But, genetics and what happens to you after you're born are the primary factors, as I understand it, of who you are and what we become." (Ibid., 1486). Note that the terms in which Judge Parslow renders his story of human development fully eclipse gestation as a meaningful, relevant, or apparently even necessary interval.

26. Dr. Justin David Call, in ibid., 918.

27. Robert A. Jones, "Another Sorry Story for Solomon," *Los Angeles Times*, September 25, 1990.

28. Martin Kasindorf, "And Baby Makes Four," *Los Angeles Times Magazine*, January 20, 1991, 33, 11, 31.

29. Trial transcript, *Johnson v. Calvert*, 914–17, 1486.

30. Cited in Dolgin, "Just a Gene," 687.

31. Pollitt, "When Is a Mother Not a Mother?" 842.

32. Neil Gotanda, "A Critique of 'Our Constitution Is Color-Blind,'" *Stanford Law Review* 44, no. 1 (1991): 1–68.

33. Lubiano, "Black Ladies," 332.

34. On the condensed meanings of the category "welfare mother," see Patricia Hill Collins, *Black Feminist Thought: Knowledge, Consciousness and the Politics of Empowerment* (New York: Routledge, 1990), 67–90; Patricia J. Williams, *The Alchemy of Race and Rights* (Cambridge: Harvard University Press, 1991); Lubiano, "Black Ladies," 323–44.

35. Toni Morrison, *Playing in the Dark: Whiteness and the Literary Imagination* (Cambridge: Harvard University Press, 1993), 21.

36. Consider a story that was carried by the Associated Press and appeared in a small local newspaper under the headline "Mother Loses Third Son to Inner-City Violence" (*Santa Cruz Sentinel*, July 9, 1993). The story itself presents a curiously confused and inconsistent picture of a woman's failed effort to protect her third and last child from the random street violence that claimed her first two sons. By her account, all of her sons did not deal drugs or carry guns and were the innocent victims of random shootings, but, according to this report, a preliminary police investigation, at least in the case of the youngest, suggested otherwise. Noting that the life expectancy of young black men is "down to less than 65 years, 10 years below the average for all Americans," the story then moves to the home of the dead son's grandmother, where relatives have gathered ostensibly to mourn. Notice, however, the way in which the scene of "mourning" is both staged and described:

Outside, barefoot kids eating grape popsicles inspected the score of quarter-size pockmarks pounded into steel security doors by the previous day's gunplay.

Inside, no tears were shed.

Mrs. Davis' sisters watched "All my Children" and braided their daughters' hair. The grandmother, 62 year-old Clara Saunders, wandered around the apartment in slippers and railed about drug dealers. (A3)

37. George J. Annas, "Crazy Making: Embryos and Gestational Mothers," *Hastings Center Report* 21, no. 1 (1991): 37.

38. Jana Sawicki, *Disciplining Foucault: Feminism, Power, and the Body* (New York: Routledge, 1991), 88.

6 / "On Breeding Good Stock": Reflections on Herrnstein and Murray's *Bell Curve*

1. Tony Perry, "San Diego Zoo Comes to the Aid of Embattled Iguana," *Los Angeles Times* (Orange County Edition), September 16, 1995, A32.

2. Ibid.

3. Richard J. Herrnstein and Charles Murray, *The Bell Curve: Intelligence and Class Structure in American Life* (New York: Free Press, 1994).

4. Ibid., 533–34.

5. In their words, "Socioeconomic status is a *result* of cognitive ability as people of high and low intelligence move to corresponding high and low places in the socioeconomic continuum." Ibid., 286.

6. Ibid., 105–15, 442. They assert also: "Inequality of endowments, including intelligence, is a reality. Trying to pretend that inequality does not really exist has led to disaster. Trying to eradicate inequality with artificially manufactured outcomes has led to disaster" (551).

7. Herrnstein and Murray give middle-class values pride of place in producing social cohesion, social order, and a civil citizenry (which, as it turns out, "a smarter population is more likely to be, and more capable of being made into"; 266). See especially 263–66.

8. Ibid., especially chaps. 13–15: "Ethnic Differences in Cognitive Ability," "Ethnic Inequalities in Relation to IQ," and "The Demography of Intelligence."

9. Karl Pearson, "On Breeding Good Stock" (1903), in *The Bell Curve Debate*, ed. Russell Jacoby and Naomi Glauberman (New York: Random House, 1994), 415.

10. Ibid., 353. They continue: "The relatively higher fertility rates of women with low IQs . . . have a larger impact on the black population as a whole than on the white."

11. Ibid., 526.

12. Ibid., 527. And earlier: "Trying to eradicate inequality with artificially manufactured outcomes has led to disaster" (551). For a general discussion of biological determinism and the political contests and confusions it has historically been deployed to resolve, see R. C. Lewontin, *Biology as Ideology* (New York: HarperCollins, 1992); R. C. Lewontin, Steven Rose, and Leon J. Kamin, *Not in Our Genes: Biology, Ideology, and Human Nature* (New York: Pantheon, 1984); Daniel J. Kevles, *In the Name of Eugenics: Genetics and the Uses of Human Heredity* (Berkeley: University of California Press, 1986); Helen E. Longino, *Science as Social Knowledge: Values and Objectivity in Scientific Inquiry* (Princeton, N.J.: Princeton University Press, 1990); Stephen Jay Gould, *The Mismeasure of Man* (New York: W. W. Norton, 1981). And from a slightly different point of view, see William Graham Sumner, *What Social Classes Owe to Each Other* (1883) (Caldwel, Idaho: Caxton, 1986).

13. Russell Jacoby and Naomi Glauberman, eds. *The Bell Curve Debate* (New York:

Random House, 1994); Steven Fraser, ed., *The Bell Curve Wars: Race, Intelligence and the Future of America* (New York: Basic Books, 1994). Let me be clear: I regard the intervention that both volumes make in the public debate over *The Bell Curve* to be important. I also find the substantial terrain that is conceded by their silence on the issue of black women's reproductive strategies to be politically troubling, dangerous, and unacceptable.

14. In both volumes there exist exceptions. See, for example, Jacqueline Jones, "Back to the Future with *The Bell Curve*: Jim Crow, Slavery, and *G*," in Fraser, *The Bell Curve Wars*, 80–93; and Alan Ryan, "Apocalypse Now?" and Ellen Willis, "The Median Is the Message," both in Jacoby and Glauberman, *The Bell Curve Debate*, 14–29 and 44–52, respectively.

15. Charles Murray, "The Coming White Underclass," *Wall Street Journal*, October 29, 1993, A14.

16. See Herrnstein and Murray, *The Bell Curve*: "Statistically, it is not good for children to be born either to a single mother or a married couple of low cognitive ability. But the greatest problems afflict children unlucky enough to be born to and reared by unmarried mothers who are also below average in intelligence—about 20 percent of the children being born. They tend to do badly, socially and economically. They tend to have low cognitive ability themselves. They suffer disproportionately from behavioral problems. They will be disproportionately represented in prisons. They are less likely to marry than others and will themselves produce large proportions of the children born to single women of low intelligence" (519). See chaps. 8 and 9 (167–201) for a discussion of the transmission of dysfunctional values and culture.

17. Ibid., 548–49.

18. Cited in Alexander Cockburn, "Norplant and the Social Cleansers, Part II," *The Nation*, July 25/August 1, 1994, 116.

19. This, at least, was how a Tulare County Superior Court judge put it on January 2, 1991, when he ordered Darlene Johnson, a black, pregnant, single parent of four, convicted of child abuse—or, in the court's words, "being a bad parent"—to be implanted with the contraceptive Norplant as a condition of her probation. In the judge's own words, "It is in the defendant's best interest and certainly *in any unconceived child's interest* that she not have any more children. . . . *Her current and unconceived children have rights, and we as a government have a duty and obligation to help these children.*" *People v. Johnson*, judgment proceedings, Tulare County Superior Court, Honorable Howard R. Broadman, presiding, January 2, 1991, 1.

20. Michael Rees, in the *New Republic*, December 9, 1991, quoted in Cockburn, "Norplant," 117. Rees is employing a notion of "children's rights" (including the right, as he renders it, not to be born into a life of hardship, or the right to be born to a certain standard of living and care) that goes back to John Stuart Mill and circulated as a compelling *moral* defense of abortion throughout the 1980s.

21. Herrnstein and Murray, *The Bell Curve*, 545.

22. Ibid.

23. Ibid., 410. For a general discussion of adoption, see 410–16.

24. Ibid.

25. Ibid., 416.

26. Ricki Solinger, *Wake Up Little Susie: Single Pregnancy and Race before Roe v. Wade* (New York: Routledge, 1992), 27.

27. Ibid., especially chaps. 1, 2.

28. As Justice Holmes put it for the Court in an opinion that permitted the forced sterilization of those regarded as feebleminded (as women who had out-of-wedlock

pregnancies typically were): "It is better for all the world, if instead of waiting to execute degenerate offspring for crime, or to let them starve for their imbecility, society can prevent those who are manifestly unfit from continuing their kind. The principle that sustains compulsory vaccination is broad enough to cover cutting the Fallopian tubes." In *The Constitutional Rights of Women: Cases in Law and Social Change*, ed. Leslie Friedman Goldstein (New York: Longman, 1979), 244. As Rosalind Petchesky points out, most of the compulsory sterilization laws from earlier in the century are still on the books. For a compelling discussion of eugenic sterilization as a strategy deployed by the state to women's sexuality as well as procreative capacity, see Petchesky's *Abortion and Woman's Choice: The State, Sexuality, and Reproductive Freedom* (New York: Longman, 1984), 67–100.

29. Solinger, *Wake Up Little Susie*, chaps. 1, 3.

30. Ibid., 17.

31. Marilyn Strathern proffers a fascinating discussion of these issues and the discourses that render an embryo/fetus outside the "natural" conjugal relationship an incomplete or deficient source of maternity or maternal identity. See "Gender: A Question of Comparison," unpublished manuscript (1992).

32. Solinger, *Wake Up Little Susie*, 77.

33. Ibid., 213. There is another story here about the development of the American welfare state and, in particular, the history of AFDC benefits that is absolutely essential to the one I am telling, but far too complex to be taken up in the context of this discussion. The literature is quite extensive, but a good beginning includes Linda Gordon, ed., *Women, the State, and Welfare* (Madison: University of Wisconsin Press, 1990); Michael B. Katz, *The Undeserving Poor: From the War on Poverty to the War on Welfare* (New York: Pantheon, 1989); Annette Lawson and Deborah L. Rhode, eds., *The Politics of Pregnancy: Adolescent Sexuality and Public Policy* (New Haven, Conn.: Yale University Press, 1993); Martha Albertson Fineman, *The Neutered Mother, the Sexual Family and Other Twentieth Century Tragedies* (New York: Routledge, 1995).

7 / Replicating the Singular Self: Some Thoughts on Cloning and Cultural Identity

1. Philip Elmer-Dewitt, "Cloning: Where Do We Draw the Line?" *Time*, November 8, 1993, 65.

2. Quoted in ibid.

3. Quoted in ibid., 69.

4. Gina Kolata, "Cloning Human Embryos," *New York Times*, October 26, 1993, A1, B7.

5. K. A. Fackelmann, "Researchers 'Clone' Human Embryos," *Science News*, October 30, 1994, 276.

6. Robert Visscher, quoted in ibid.

7. Leon R. Kass, "The New Biology: What Price Relieving Man's Estate?" *Science* 174 (1971): 779.

8. Arnold I. Davidson develops a provocative analysis of these themes in "The Horror of Monsters," in *The Boundaries of Humanity: Humans, Animals, Machines*, ed. James J. Sheehan and Morton Sosna (Berkeley: University of California Press, 1991), 36–67. On the anxieties, fears, and arrogance that have shaped the development of the (reproductive) life sciences in the United States over the course of the past century, see

Adele E. Clarke, *Disciplining Reproduction: Modernity, American Life Sciences, and the "Problem of Sex"* (Berkeley: University of California Press, forthcoming).

9. Albert Rosenfeld, "Science, Sex, and Tomorrow's Morality," *Life*, June 13, 1969, 38–54.

10. David M. Rorvik, "Taking Life in Our Own Hands: The Test-Tube Baby Is Coming," *Life*, May 18, 1971, 88.

11. Sarah Franklin, "Postmodern Procreation: A Cultural Account of Assisted Reproduction," in *Conceiving the New World Order: The Global Politics of Reproduction*, ed. Faye D. Ginsberg and Rayna Rapp (Berkeley: University of California Press, 1995); see also Marilyn Strathern, *After Nature: English Kinship in the Late Twentieth Century* (Cambridge: Cambridge University Press, 1992).

12. Sarah Franklin, "Essentialism, Which Essentialism? Some Implications of Reproductive and Genetic Techno-Science," *Journal of Homosexuality* 24, nos. 3–4 (1993): 29.

13. For a provocative reading on global fertility struggles and strategies, see Donna Haraway, "Virtual Speculum in the New World Order," in *Modern Witness@Second Millennium. FemaleMan© Meets OncoMouse™* (New York: Routledge, forthcoming).

14. Quoted in Elmer-Dewitt, "Cloning," 67, 70.

15. Robert Blank, *The Political Implications of Human Genetic Technology* (Boulder, Colo.: Westview, 1981).

16. About my use of the terms *autonomy* and *agency:* At this juncture in the argument, I mean to invoke the conventional meanings and understandings of these practices (and the subject they conjure) insofar as conventional renderings—although not unproblematic—are nevertheless what shape and are seen as being at stake in the public controversy over cloning.

17. Mary Douglas, *How Institutions Think* (Syracuse, N.Y.: Syracuse University Press, 1986), 63, 92.

18. Donna Haraway, "The Biopolitics of Postmodern Bodies: Constitutions of Self in Immune System Discourse," in *Simians, Cyborgs, and Women: The Reinvention of Nature* (New York: Routledge, 1991), 203–30.

19. Evelynn Hammonds, "Black (W)holes and the Geometry of Black Female Sexuality," *differences* 6, nos. 2–3 (1994): 126–45.

20. Diane B. Paul, "Eugenic Anxieties, Social Realities, and the Genome Initiative," paper presented at the "Genes R Us" conference, Humanities Research Institute, University of California, Irvine, 1993, 1. A revised version of this paper was published as "Eugenic Anxieties, Social Realities, and Political Choices," in *Are Genes Us? The Social Consequences of the New Genetics*, ed. Carl F. Cranor (New Brunswick, N.J.: Rutgers University Press, 1994), 142–54. See also Andrew Kimbrell, *The Human Body Shop: The Engineering and Marketing of Life* (New York: HarperCollins, 1993).

21. Paul, "Eugenic Anxieties," 1.

22. Elmer-Dewitt, "Cloning," 65, 69.

23. Richard J. Herrnstein and Charles Murray, *The Bell Curve: Intelligence and Class Structure in American Life* (New York: Free Press, 1994), see especially 1–24.

24. Kolata, "Cloning Human Embryos," B7; Elmer-Dewitt, "Cloning," 68.

25. Saidiya Hartman, "Seduction and the Ruses of Power," unpublished manuscript (1992); Patricia J. Williams, "On Being the Object of Property," in *The Alchemy of Race and Rights* (Cambridge: Harvard University Press, 1991), 216–38; Cheryl I. Harris, "Whiteness as Property," *Harvard Law Review* 106 (1993): 1707–91.

26. What is interesting is that once their intentions were made public, other couples came forward to disclose that they too had conceived for similar reasons.

27. For a provocative reading of *John Moore v. the Regents of the University of California,* see Paul Rabinow, "Severing the Ties: Fragmentation and Dignity in Late Modernity," in *Essays in the Anthropology of Reason* (Princeton, N.J.: Princeton University Press, 1996).

28. "It was clear that it was just a matter of time until someone was going to do it, and we decided it would be better for us to do it in an open manner and get the ethical questions moving." Quoted in Rebecca Kolberg, "Human Embryo Cloning Reported," *Science,* October 29, 1993, 652.

29. Leon Kass, "Making Babies: The New Biology and the 'Old' Morality," *Public Interest* 26 (Winter 1972): 42–44.

30. Arthur Caplan, quoted in Kolata, "Cloning Human Embryos," B7.

31. One hears and reads increasingly of sperm being extracted from corpses at the request of family members. I am thinking here, in particular, of a couple who within weeks of being married were in a car wreck. The man died. At the hospital, his father urged the doctors to salvage sperm from the corpse so that his daughter-in-law could later be inseminated. The idea was that his son would then live on through the birth of a child. About how his widow felt, we can only speculate.

32. Arthus Caplan, quoted in Kolata, "Cloning Human Embryos," B7.

33. Ibid.

34. Ibid.

35. Quoted in Elmer-Dewitt, "Cloning," 69.

36. Office of Technology Assessment, "Do Property Rights Adhere to Individuals or the Species?" in *Biology, Medicine, and the Bill of Rights* (Washington, D.C.: U.S. Government Printing Office, 1988), 23.

37. George J. Annas, "Crazy Making: Embryos and Gestational Mothers," *Hastings Center Report* 21, no. 1 (1991): 37.

38. Franklin makes this distinction in "Postmodern Procreation." See also Evelyn Fox Keller, "From Secrets of Life to Secrets of Death," in *Secrets of Life, Secrets of Death: Essays on Language, Gender, and Science* (New York: Routledge, 1992), 39–55.

39. Sarah Franklin, "Fetal Fascinations: New Dimensions to the Medical-Scientific Construction of Fetal Personhood," in *Off-Centre: Feminism and Cultural Studies,* ed. Sarah Franklin, Celia Lury, and Jackie Stacey (New York: HarperCollins, 1991), 193.

40. A. L. R. Findley, *Reproduction and the Fetus* (London: Edward Arnold, 1984), 83, quoted in ibid., 194.

41. Listen to the account of fetal life, or what Franklin in "Fetal Fascinations" characterizes as "the new 'natural facts' of pregnancy," proffered by one fetologist, but certainly echoed, enthusiastically, by others: "The fetus is thought of nowadays not as an inert passenger in pregnancy but, rather, as in command of it. The fetus, in collaboration with the placenta, (a) ensures the endocrine success of pregnancy, (b) induces changes in maternal physiology which make her a suitable host, (c) is responsible for solving the immunological problems raised by its intimate contact with its mother, and (d) determines the duration of pregnancy." Findley, *Reproduction and the Fetus,* 96, quoted in Franklin, "Fetal Fascintions," 193.

42. Walter Gilbert, "A Vision of the Grail," in *The Code of Codes: Scientific and Social Issues in the Human Genome Project,* ed. Daniel J. Kevles and Leroy Hood (Cambridge: Harvard University Press, 1992), 93.

43. Ibid.

44. As Evelyn Fox Keller points out, how these practices might be refigured is itself a thoroughly vexing question. In Keller's words: "Today we are being told—and judging from media accounts, we are apparently coming to believe—that what makes us human

is our genes. Indeed, the very notion of 'culture' as distinct from 'biology' seems to have vanished; in terms that increasingly dominate contemporary discourse, 'culture' has become subsumed under biology. . . . But if culture is to be subsumed under biology, and if it is our biological or genetic future that we now seek to shape, where are we to locate the domain of freedom by which this future can be charted? The disarming suggestion that is put forth is that this domain of freedom is to be found in the elusive realm of 'individual choice'—a suggestion that invokes a democratic and egalitarian ideal somewhere beyond biology. But since there is in this discourse no domain 'beyond biology,' since it is our genes that 'make us what we are,' and since they do so with definitive inequality that compromises even those choices some of us can make, we are obliged to look elsewhere for the implied realm of freedom." "Nature, Nurture, and the Human Genome Project," in *The Code of Codes: Scientific and Social Issues in the Human Genome Project*, ed. Daniel J. Kevles and Leroy Hood (Cambridge: Harvard University Press, 1992), 297–98.

45. As Evelyn Fox Keller observes, "Molecular geneticists do not seek genetic loci for traits that they—and we—accept as *normal*." Ibid., 298. Or, as Dorothy Nelkin and M. Susan Lindee put the matter: "People with problems [will] become, in effect, problem people." *The DNA Mystique: The Gene as a Cultural Icon* (New York: W. H. Freeman, 1995), 129. See also Dorothy Nelkin, "The Social Power of Genetic Information," in *The Code of Codes: Scientific and Social Issues in the Human Genome Project*, ed. Daniel J. Kevles and Leroy Hood (Cambridge: Harvard University Press, 1992): "As has often been the case in the history of medical intervention, diagnostic techniques are far ahead of therapeutic possibilities. For the short term, perhaps the most important social consequence of these new diagnostic tests will arise less from their actual use than from their bearing on the definition of deviance and disease" (179).

46. Katharine T. Bartlett, "Re-expressing Parenthood," *Yale Law Journal* 98 (1988): 295.

47. Brief amicus curiae of the American Civil Liberties Union of Southern California, Jon W. Davidson and Paul L. Hoffman (August 1991); brief amicus curiae of the American Civil Liberties Union of Southern California, Jon W. Davidson, Carol A. Sobel, and Paul L. Hoffman (December 1992).

48. See, for example, Gena Corea, *The Mother Machine: Reproductive Technologies from Artificial Insemination to Artificial Wombs* (New York: Harper & Row, 1985); Patricia Spallone and Deborah Lynn Steinberg, eds., *Made to Order: The Myth of Reproductive and Genetic Progress* (New York: Pergamon, 1987).

49. Quoted in Kolata, "Cloning Human Embryos," B7.

Bibliography

Aeschylus. 1953. *Oresteia*, trans. Richard Lattimore. Chicago: University of Chicago Press.

Andrews, Lori B. 1986. "My Body My Property." *Hastings Center Report* 16 (5): 28–38.

———. 1987. "The Aftermath of Baby M: Proposed State Laws on Surrogate Motherhood." *Hastings Center Report* 17 (5): 31–40.

Annas, George J. 1986. "Pregnant Women as Fetal Containers." *Hastings Center Report* 16 (6): 13–14.

———. 1987. "Baby M: Babies and Justice for Sale." *Hastings Center Report* 17 (3): 13–15.

———. 1991. "Crazy Making: Embryos and Gestational Mothers." *Hastings Center Report* 21 (1): 35–38.

Annas, George J., and Sherman Elias, eds. 1992. *Gene Mapping: Using Law and Ethics as Guides*. New York: Oxford University Press.

Aristotle. 1979. *Generation of Animals*, trans. A. L. Peck. Cambridge: Harvard University Press.

Armstrong, David. 1983. *Political Anatomy of the Body: Medical Knowledge in the Twentieth Century*. Cambridge: Cambridge University Press.

Arnold, Regina. 1990. "Processes of Victimization and Criminalization of Black Women." *Social Justice* 17 (3): 153–66.

Aronowitz, Stanley. 1988. *Science as Power: Discourse and Ideology in Modern Society*. Minneapolis: University of Minnesota Press.

"Baby M," Supreme Court of New Jersey, 537 A.2D at 1277 (1988).

Baker, Dan. 1985. *Beyond Choice: The Abortion Story No One Is Telling*. Portland, Ore.: Multnomah.

Balsamo, Anne. 1996. *Technologies of the Gendered Body: Reading Cyborg Women*. Durham: Duke University Press.

157

Barnouw, Dagmar. 1995. "Seeing and Believing: The Thin Blue Line of Documentary Objectivity." *Common Knowledge* 4 (1): 129–43.

Bartlett, Katharine T. 1988. "Re-expressing Parenthood" *Yale Law Journal* 98: 293–340.

Bartlett, Katharine T., and Rosanne Kennedy, eds. 1991. *Feminist Legal Theory: Readings in Law and Gender*. Boulder, Colo.: Westview.

Baruch, Elaine Hoffman, Amadeo F. D'Adamo Jr., and Joni Seager, eds. 1988. *Embryos, Ethics, and Women's Rights: Exploring the New Reproductive Technologies*. New York: Harrington Park.

Bassin, Donna, ed., with Margaret Honey and Meryle Mahrer Kaplan. 1994. *Representations of Motherhood*. New Haven, Conn.: Yale University Press.

Bayles, Michael D. 1984. *Reproductive Ethics*. Englewood Cliffs, N.J.: Prentice Hall.

Begley, Sharon. 1995. "Infertility: Has the Hype Outweighed the Hope?" *Newsweek,* September 4, 38–45.

Begley, Sharon, with Mary Hager, Daniel Glick, and Jennifer Foote. 1993. "Cures from the Womb." *Newsweek,* February 22, 49–51.

Bennett, Neil G., ed. 1983. *Sex Selection of Children*. New York: Harcourt Brace Jovanovich.

Blank, Robert. 1981. *The Political Implications of Human Genetic Technology*. Boulder, Colo.: Westview.

———. 1988. "The Changing Nature of Human Nature: DNA Probes and the Human Genome." Unpublished manuscript.

———. 1990. *Regulating Reproduction*. New York: Columbia University Press.

Bondeson, William B., H. Tristram Engelhardt Jr., Stuart F. Spicker, and Daniel H. Winship, eds. 1984. *Abortion and the Status of the Fetus*. Boston: D. Reidel.

Bray v. Alexandria Women's Health Clinic, 113 S.Ct. 753 (1993).

Butler, J. Douglas, and David F. Walbert, eds., 1986. *Abortion, Medicine and the Law*. New York: Facts on File.

Butler, Judith. 1993. "Endangered/Endangering: Schematic Racism and White Paranoia." In *Reading Rodney King, Reading Urban Uprising*, ed. Robert Gooding-Williams. New York: Routledge.

Butler, Judith, and Joan W. Scott. 1992. *Feminists Theorize the Political*. New York: Routledge.

Canguilhem, George. 1991. *On the Normal and the Pathological*, trans. Carolyn R. Fawcett. New York: Zone.

Casper, Monica J. 1995. "Fetal Cyborgs and Technomoms on the Reproductive Frontier: Which Way to the Carnival?" In *The Cyborg Handbook*, ed. Chris Hables Gray with Heidi J. Figueroa-Sarriera and Steven Mentor. New York: Routledge.

Clarke, Adele E. 1995. "Modernity, Postmodernity, and Reproductive Processes, ca. 1890–1990, or 'Mommy, Where Do Cyborgs Come from Anyway?'" In *The Cyborg Handbook*, ed. Chris Hables Gray with Heidi J. Figueroa-Sarriera and Steven Mentor. New York: Routledge.

———. forthcoming. *Disciplining Reproduction: Modernity, American Life Sciences, and the "Problem of Sex."* Berkeley: University of California Press.

Clayton, Raymond. 1983. "The Biomedical Revolution and Totalitarian Control." In *On Nineteen Eighty-Four*, ed. Peter Stansky. New York: W. H. Freeman.

Cockburn, Alexander. 1994. "Norplant and the Social Cleansers, Part II." *The Nation,* July 25/August 1.

Cohen, Sherrill, and Nadine Taub, eds. 1989. *Reproductive Laws for the 1990s*. Clifton, N.J.: Humana.

Collins, Patricia Hill. 1990. *Black Feminist Thought: Knowledge, Consciousness and the Politics of Empowerment*. New York: Routledge.

Condit, Michelle. 1990. *Decoding Abortion Rhetoric: Communicating Social Change*. Chicago: University of Illinois Press.

Corea, Gena. 1985. *The Mother Machine: Reproductive Technologies from Artificial Insemination to Artificial Wombs*. New York: Harper & Row.

Cranor, Carl F. 1994. *Are Genes Us? The Social Consequences of the New Genetics*. New Brunswick, N.J.: Rutgers University Press.

Crary, Jonathan. 1995. *Techniques of the Observer: On Vision and Modernity in the Nineteenth Century*. Cambridge: MIT Press.

Crary, Jonathan, and Sanford Kwinter, eds. 1992. *Incorporations*. New York: Zone.

Crenshaw, Kimberlé, and Gary Peller. 1993. "Reel Time/Real Justice." In *Reading Rodney King, Reading Urban Uprising*, ed. Robert Gooding-Williams. New York: Routledge.

Daniels, Cynthia R. 1993. *At Women's Expense: State Power and the Politics of Fetal Rights*. Cambridge: Harvard University Press.

Daston, Lorraine, and Peter Galison. 1992. "The Image of Objectivity." *Representations* 40: 81–128.

Davidson, Arnold I. 1991. "The Horror of Monsters." In *The Boundaries of Humanity: Humans, Animals, Machines*, ed. James J. Sheehan and Morton Sosna. Berkeley: University of California Press.

Davies, Susan E., ed. 1988. *Women under Attack: Victories, Backlash and the Fight for Reproductive Freedom*, Pamphlet 7, Committee for Abortion Rights and Against Sterilization Abuse. Boston: South End.

de Lauretis, Teresa. 1987. *Technologies of Gender*. Bloomington: Indiana University Press.

Delaney, Carol. 1986. "The Meaning of Paternity and the Virgin Birth Debate." *Man* 21: 494–513.

D'Emilio, John, and Estelle B. Freedman. 1988. *Intimate Matters: A History of Sexuality in America*. New York: Harper & Row.

Doane, Janice, and Devon Hodges. 1989. "Risky Business: Familial Ideology and the Case of Baby M." *differences* 1 (1): 67–81.

Dolgin, Janet L. 1990. "Status and Contract in Surrogate Motherhood: An Illumination of the Surrogacy Debate." *Buffalo Law Review* 38: 515–50.

———. 1992. "Family Law and the Facts of Family." Unpublished manuscript.

———. 1993. "Just a Gene: Judicial Assumptions about Parenthood." *UCLA Law Review* 40: 637–94.

Douglas, Mary. 1986. *How Institutions Think*. Syracuse, N.Y.: Syracuse University Press.

Drakich, Janice. 1989. "In Search of the Better Parent: The Social Construction of Ideologies of Fatherhood." *Canadian Journal of Women and the Law* 3: 69–87.

Dreyfus, Hubert L., and Paul Rabinow. 1983. *Michel Foucault: Beyond Structuralism and Hermeneutics*. Chicago: University of Chicago Press.

Duden, Barbara. 1993. *Disembodying Women: Perspectives on Pregnancy and the Unborn*, trans. Lee Hoinacki. Cambridge: Harvard University Press.

Duster, Troy. 1990. *Backdoor to Eugenics*. New York: Routledge.

Dworkin, Ronald. 1994. *Life's Dominion: An Argument about Abortion, Euthanasia, and Individual Freedom*. New York: Vintage.

Dyer, Richard. 1993. *The Matter of Images: Essays on Representations*. London: Routledge.

Edwards, Jeanette, Sarah Franklin, Eric Hirsch, Francis Price, and Marilyn Strathern. 1993. *Technologies of Procreation: Kinship in the Age of Assisted Conception.* Manchester: Manchester University Press.

Eisenstein, Zillah. 1982. "The Sexual Politics of the New Right: The 'Crisis of Liberalism' for the 1980s." *Signs* 7: 567–88.

———. 1988. *The Female Body and the Law.* Berkeley: University of California Press.

Elmer-Dewitt, Philip. 1991. "Curing Infertility: Making Babies." *Time,* September 30, 56–63.

———. 1993. "Cloning: Where Do We Draw the Line?" *Time,* November 8, 65–70.

Elshtain, Jean Bethke, ed. 1982. *The Family in Political Thought.* Amherst: University of Massachusetts Press.

Euripides. 1958. *The Bacchae,* trans. William Arrowsmith. Chicago: University of Chicago Press.

Faludi, Susan. 1991. *Backlash: The Undeclared War against American Women.* New York: Anchor.

Fineman, Martha Albertson. 1995. *The Neutered Mother, the Sexual Family and Other Twentieth Century Tragedies.* New York: Routledge.

Fineman, Martha Albertson, and Nancy Sweet Thomadsen, eds. 1991. *At the Boundaries of Law: Feminism and Legal Theory.* New York: Routledge.

Fletcher, Joseph C., and Mark I. Evans. 1983. "Maternal Bonding in Early Fetal Ultrasound Examinations." *New England Journal of Medicine* 308: 392–93.

Foucault, Michel. 1980. *The History of Sexuality,* vol. 1. New York: Vintage.

———. 1980. *Power/Knowledge; Selected Interviews and Other Writings,* ed. and trans. Colin Gordon. New York: Pantheon.

Franklin, Sarah. 1990. "Deconstructing 'Desperateness': The Social Construction of Infertility in Popular Representations of New Reproductive Technologies." In *The New Reproductive Technologies,* ed. Maureen McNeil, Ian Varcoe, and Steven Yearly. London: Macmillan.

———. 1991. "Fetal Fascinations: New Dimensions to the Medical-Scientific Construction of Fetal Personhood." In *Off-Centre: Feminism and Cultural Studies,* ed. Sarah Franklin, Celia Lury, and Jackie Stacey. New York: HarperCollins.

———. 1993. "Essentialism, Which Essentialism? Some Implications of Reproductive and Genetic Techno-Science." *Journal of Homosexuality* 24, nos. 3–4 (1993): 27–40.

———1995. "Postmodern Procreation: A Cultural Account of Assisted Reproduction." In *Conceiving the New World Order: The Global Politics of Reproduction,* ed. Faye D. Ginsberg and Rayna Rapp. Berkeley: University of California Press.

———.1995. "Romancing the Helix: Nature and Scientific Discovery." In *Romancing Revisited,* ed. L. Pearce and J. Stacey. London: Falmer.

Franklin, Sarah, Celia Lury, and Jackie Stacey, eds. 1991. *Off-Centre: Feminism and Cultural Studies.* New York: HarperCollins.

Fraser, Nancy. 1989. *Unruly Practices: Power, Discourse, and Gender in Contemporary Social Theory.* Minneapolis: University of Minnesota Press.

Fraser, Steven, ed. 1994. *The Bell Curve Wars: Race, Intelligence and the Future of America.* New York: Basic Books.

Fried, Marlene Gerber, ed. 1990. *From Abortion to Reproductive Freedom: Transforming a Movement.* Boston: South End.

Fuchs, Cynthia J. 1993. "'Death is Irrelevant': Cyborgs, Reproduction, and the Future of Male Hysteria." *Genders* 18: 113–33.

Fuss, Diana, ed. 1996. *Human, All Too Human.* New York: Routledge.

Gaines, Jane M. 1991. *Contested Culture: The Image, the Voice, and the Law*. Chapel Hill: University of North Carolina Press.

Gaines, Jane M., and Charlotte Herzog, eds. 1990. *Fabrications: Costume and the Female Body*. New York: Routledge.

Gallagher, Janet. 1985. "Fetal Personhood and Women's Policy." In *Women, Biology, and Public Policy*, ed. Virginia Sapiro. Beverly Hills: Sage.

―――. 1987. "Prenatal Invasions and Interventions: What's Wrong with Fetal Rights." *Harvard Women's Law Journal* 10: 9–58.

Garb, Maggie. 1989. "Abortion Foes Give Birth to a 'Syndrome.'" *In These Times*, February 22–March 1.

Garfield, Jay L., and Patricia Hennessey, eds. 1984. *Abortion: Moral and Legal Perspectives*. Amherst: University of Massachusetts Press.

Garrow, David J. 1994. *Liberty and Sexuality: The Right to Privacy and the Making of Roe v. Wade*. New York: Macmillan.

Geertz, Clifford. 1983. *Local Knowledge: Further Essays in Interpretive Anthropology*. New York: Basic Books.

Gerson, Deborah. 1989. "Infertility and the Construction of Desperation." *Socialist Review* 19 (3): 45–64.

Gibbs, Nancy. 1989. "Want a Baby?" *Time*, October 9, 86–89.

Gilbert, Walter. 1992. "A Vision of the Grail." In *The Code of Codes: Scientific and Social Issues in the Human Genome Project*, ed. Daniel J. Kevles and Leroy Hood. Cambridge: Harvard University Press.

Ginsberg, Faye D. 1989. *Contested Lives: The Abortion Debate in an American Community*. Berkeley: University of California Press.

Ginsberg, Faye D., and Rayna Rapp, eds. 1995. *Conceiving the New World Order: The Global Politics of Reproduction*. Berkeley: University of California Press.

Ginsberg, Faye D., and Anna Lowenhaupt Tsing, eds. 1990. *Uncertain Terms: Negotiating Gender in American Culture*. Boston: Beacon.

Glendon, Mary Ann. 1987. *Abortion and Divorce in Western Law*. Cambridge: Harvard University Press.

Goldberg, David Theo. 1993. *Racist Culture: Philosophy and the Politics of Meaning*. Cambridge, Mass.: Blackwell.

Goldberg, James D., ed. 1993. "Fetal Medicine" (special issue). *Western Journal of Medicine* 159 (3).

Goldstein, Leslie Friedman, ed. 1979. *The Constitutional Rights of Women: Cases in Law and Social Change*. New York: Longman.

Gooding-Williams, Robert, ed. 1993. *Reading Rodney King, Reading Urban Uprising*. New York: Routledge.

Gordon, Linda, ed. 1990. *Women, the State, and Welfare*. Madison: University of Wisconsin Press.

Gostin, Larry, ed. 1990. *Surrogate Motherhood: Politics and Privacy*. Bloomington: Indiana University Press.

Gotanda, Neil. 1991. "A Critique of 'Our Constitution Is Color-Blind.'" *Stanford Law Review* 44: 1–68.

Gould, Stephen Jay. 1981. *The Mismeasure of Man*. New York: W. W. Norton.

Gray, Chris Hables, ed., with Heidi J. Figueroa-Sarriera and Steven Mentor. 1995. *The Cyborg Handbook*. New York: Routledge.

Hammonds, Evelynn. 1994. "Black (W)holes and the Geometry of Black Female Sexuality." *differences* 6 (2–3): 126–45.

Haraway, Donna. 1990. "Investment Strategies for the Evolving Portfolio of Primate

Females." In *Body/Politics: Women and the Discourses of Science*, ed. Mary Jacobus, Evelyn Fox Keller, and Sally Shuttleworth. New York: Routledge.

———. 1991. *Simians, Cyborgs, and Women: The Reinvention of Nature*. New York: Routledge.

———. 1992. "The Promise of Monsters: A Regenerative Politics for Inappropriate/d Others." In *Cultural Studies*, ed. Lawrence Grossberg, Cary Nelson, and Paula A. Treichler. New York: Routledge.

———. forthcoming. *Modern Witness@Second Millennium. FemaleMan© Meets OncoMouse™*. New York: Routledge.

Harding, Sandra, and Jean F. O'Barr, eds. 1987. *Sex and Scientific Inquiry*. Chicago: University of Chicago Press.

Harding, Susan. 1990. "If I Should Die before I Wake: Jerry Falwell's Pro-Life Gospel." In *Uncertain Terms: Negotiating Gender in American Culture*, ed. Faye D. Ginsberg and Anna Lowenhaupt Tsing. Boston: Beacon.

Harris, Cheryl I. 1993. "Whiteness as Property." *Harvard Law Review* 106: 1707–91.

Hartman, Saidiya. 1992. "Seduction and the Ruses of Power." Unpublished manuscript.

Hartouni, Valerie. 1993. "*Brave New World* in the Discourses of Reproductive and Genetic Technologies." In *In the Nature of Things: Language, Politics, and the Environment*, ed. Jane Bennett and William Chaloupka. Minneapolis: University of Minnesota Press.

Hayler, Barbara. 1979. "Review Essay: Abortion." *Signs* 4: 322–33.

Herrnstein, Richard J., and Charles Murray. 1994. *The Bell Curve: Intelligence and Class Structure in American Life*. New York: Free Press.

Hobbes, Thomas. 1974. *Leviathan*, ed. Michael Oakeshott. New York: Collier.

Holmes, Helen Bequaert, ed. 1992. *Issues in Reproductive Technology: An Anthology*. New York: Garland.

Holmes, Helen Bequaert, Betty B. Hoskins, and Michael Gross, eds. 1981. *The Custom-Made Child: Women-Centered Perspectives*. Clifton, N.J.: Humana.

Horn, David G. 1994. *Social Bodies: Science Reproduction and Italian Modernity*. Princeton, N.J.: Princeton University Press.

Hubbard, Ruth. 1984. "Personal Courage Is Not Enough: Some Hazards of Childbearing in the 1980s." In *Test-Tube Women*, ed. Rita Arditti, Renate Duelli Klein, and Shelly Minden. Boston: Pandora.

———. 1992. *The Politics of Women's Biology*. New Brunswick, N.J.: Rutgers University Press.

Hubbard, Ruth, and Elijah Wald. 1993. *Exploding the Gene Myth*. Boston: Beacon.

Hunter, Nan. 1983. "State Legislation Concerning 'Feticide' and 'Wrongful Birth/Wrongful Life,'" Memorandum to ACLU Affiliates, Reproductive Freedom Project (April 15).

———. 1986. "Feticide: Cases and Legislation." Memorandum to the ACLU, Reproductive Freedom Project (May 5).

Huxley, Aldous. 1946. *Brave New World*. New York: Harper & Row.

———. 1958. *Brave New World Revisited*. New York: Harper & Brothers.

Jacobsohn, Gary. 1986. *The Supreme Court and the Decline of Constitutional Aspiration*. Totowa, N.J.: Rowman & Littlefield.

Jacobus, Mary, Evelyn Fox Keller, and Sally Shuttleworth, eds. 1990. *Body/Politics: Women and the Discourses of Science*. New York: Routledge.

Jacoby, Russell, and Naomi Glauberman, eds. 1994. *The Bell Curve Debate*. New York: Random House.

Jaroff, Leon. 1989. "Solving the Mysteries of Heredity." *Time*, March 20, 62–67.

Jenks, Chris, ed. 1995. *Visual Culture*. London: Routledge.

Johnsen, Dawn E. 1986. "The Creation of Fetal Rights: Conflicts with Women's Constitutional Rights to Liberty, Privacy, and Equal Protection." *Yale Law Journal* 95: 599–625.

Johnson v. Calvert. 1990. Transcript, Office of the Supreme Court, California.

Kairys, David, ed. 1982. *The Politics of Law: A Progressive Critique*. New York: Pantheon.

Kaplan, E. Ann. 1992. *Motherhood and Representation: The Mother in Popular Culture and Melodrama*. New York: Routledge.

Kass, Leon R. 1971. "The New Biology: What Price Relieving Man's Estate?" *Science* 174: 779–88.

———. 1972. "Making Babies: The New Biology and the 'Old' Morality." *Public Interest* 26: 16–56.

———. 1979. "Making Babies Revisited." *Public Interest* 54: 32–60.

Katz, Michael B. 1989. *The Undeserving Poor: From the War on Poverty to the War on Welfare*. New York: Pantheon.

Keller, Evelyn Fox. 1985. *Reflections on Gender and Science*. New Haven, Conn.: Yale University Press.

———. 1992. "Nature, Nurture, and the Human Genome Project." In *The Code of Codes: Scientific and Social Issues in the Human Genome Project*, ed. Daniel J. Kevles and Leroy Hood. Cambridge: Harvard University Press.

———. 1992. *Secrets of Life, Secrets of Death: Essays on Language, Gender and Science*. New York: Routledge.

Kenney, Sally J. 1992. *For Whose Protection? Reproductive Hazards and Exclusionary Policies in the United States and Britain*. Ann Arbor: University of Michigan Press.

Kevles, Daniel J. 1986. *In the Name of Eugenics: Genetics and the Uses of Human Heredity*. Berkeley: University of California Press.

———. 1995. "Genetics, Race, and IQ: From Binet to *The Bell Curve*." *Contention: Debates in Society, Culture, and Science* 5 (1): 3–18.

Kevles, Daniel J., and Leroy Hood, eds. 1992. *The Code of Codes: Scientific and Social Issues in the Human Genome Project*. Cambridge: Harvard University Press.

Kimbrell, Andrew. 1993. *The Human Body Shop: The Engineering and Marketing of Life*. New York: HarperCollins.

Knorr-Cetina, Karen, and Michael Mulkey. 1983. *Science Observed: Perspectives on the Social Study of Science*. Beverly Hills: Sage.

Lake, Randell A. 1986. "The Metaethical Framework of Anti-Abortion Rhetoric." *Signs* 11: 478–99.

Laqueur, Thomas W. 1990. "The Facts of Fatherhood." In *Conflicts in Feminism*, ed. Marianne Hirsch and Evelyn Fox Keller. New York: Routledge.

———. 1990. *Making Sex: Body and Gender from the Greeks to Freud*. Cambridge: Harvard University Press.

Latour, Bruno. 1987. *Science in Action*. Cambridge: Harvard University Press.

———. 1994. *We Have Never Been Modern*, trans. Catherine Porter. Cambridge: Harvard University Press.

Latour, Bruno, and Steve Woolgar. 1986. *Laboratory Life: The Social Construction of Scientific Facts*. Princeton, N.J.: Princeton University Press.

Lawson, Annette, and Deborah L. Rhode, eds. 1993. *The Politics of Pregnancy: Adolescent Sexuality and Public Policy*. New Haven, Conn.: Yale University Press.

Layne, Linda L. 1992. "Of Fetuses and Angels: Fragmentation and Integration in Narratives of Pregnancy Loss." *Knowledge and Society: The Anthropology of Science and Technology* 9: 29–58.

Le Goff, Jacques. 1988. "Head or Heart? The Political Use of Body Metaphors in the Middle Ages." In *Fragments for a History of the Human Body*, ed. Michael Feher with Romina Naddaff and Nadia Tazi. New York: Zone.

Lewontin, R. C. 1992. *Biology as Ideology*. New York: HarperCollins.

Lewontin, R. C., Steven Rose, and Leon J. Kamin. 1984. *Not in Our Genes: Biology, Ideology, and Human Nature*. New York: Pantheon.

Lloyd, G. E. R., ed. 1978. *Hippocratic Writings*, trans. J. Chadwick and W. N. Mann. New York: Penguin.

Lloyd, Genevieve. 1984. *The Man of Reason: "Male" and "Female" in Western Philosophy*. Minneapolis: University of Minnesota Press.

Locke, John. 1963. *Two Treatises of Government*, ed. Peter Laslett. New York: New American Library.

Longino, Helen E. 1990. *Science as Social Knowledge: Values and Objectivity in Scientific Inquiry*. Princeton, N.J.: Princeton University Press.

Lubiano, Wahneema. 1992. "Black Ladies, Welfare Queens, and State Minstrels: Ideological War by Narrative Means." In *Race-ing Justice, En-gendering Power: Essays on Anita Hill, Clarence Thomas, and the Construction of Social Reality*, ed. Toni Morrison. New York: Pantheon.

Luker, Kristen. 1984. *Abortion and the Politics of Motherhood*. Berkeley: University of California Press.

Macklin, Ruth. 1991. "Artificial Means of Reproduction and Our Understanding of the Family." *Hastings Center Report* 21 (1): 5–11.

Macpherson, C. B. 1962. *The Political Theory of Possessive Individualism*. Oxford: Oxford University Press.

Maher, Lisa. 1990. "Criminalizing Pregnancy: The Downside of a Kinder, Gentler Nation?" *Social Justice* 17 (3): 111–35.

Manoff, Robert Karl, and Michael Schudson, eds. 1986. *Reading the News*. New York: Pantheon.

Marcuse, Herbert. 1964. *One-Dimensional Man*. Boston: Beacon.

Martin, Emily. 1987. *The Woman in the Body: A Cultural Analysis of Reproduction*. Boston: Beacon.

———. 1990. "The Ideology of Reproduction and the Reproduction of Ideology." In *Uncertain Terms: Negotiating Gender in American Culture*, ed. Faye D. Ginsberg and Anna Lowenhaupt Tsing. Boston: Beacon.

———. 1991. "The Egg and Sperm." *Signs* 16: 485–501.

Mason, Steven. 1968. *A History of the Sciences*. New York: Collier.

McNeil, Maureen, and Sarah Franklin. 1991. "Science and Technology: Questions for Cultural Studies and Feminism." In *Off-Centre: Feminism and Cultural Studies*, ed. Sarah Franklin, Celia Lury, and Jackie Stacey. New York: HarperCollins.

McNeil, Maureen, Ian Varcoe, and Steven Yearley, eds. 1990. *The New Reproductive Technologies*. London: Macmillan.

Mercer, Kobena. 1994. *Welcome to the Jungle: New Positions in Black Cultural Studies*. New York: Routledge.

Mill, John Stuart. 1980. *The Subjection of Women*, ed. Sue Mansfield. Arlington Heights, Ill.: Harlan Davidson.

Minow, Martha. 1990. *Making All the Difference: Inclusion, Exclusion, and American Law*. Ithaca, N.Y.: Cornell University Press.

Minow, Martha, Michael Ryan, and Austin Sarat, eds. 1992. *Narrative, Violence, and the Law: The Essays of Robert Cover*. Ann Arbor: University of Michigan Press.

Mitchell, W. J. T. 1986. *Iconology: Image, Text, Ideology*. Chicago: University of Chicago Press.

Mohr, James C. 1978. *Abortion in America: The Origins and Evolution of National Policy*. New York: Oxford University Press.

Montrose, Louis. 1991. "The Work of Gender in the Discourse of Discovery." *Representations* 33: 1–41.

Moon, Donald J. 1993. *Constructing Community: Moral Pluralism and Tragic Conflicts*. Princeton, N.J.: Princeton University Press.

Morrison, Toni, ed. 1992. *Race-ing Justice, En-gendering Power: Essays on Anita Hill, Clarence Thomas, and the Construction of Social Reality*. New York: Pantheon.

———. 1993. *Playing in the Dark: Whiteness and the Literary Imagination*. Cambridge: Harvard University Press.

Murray, Charles. 1992. "Stop Favoring Unwed Mothers." *New York Times*, January 16, A23.

———. 1993. "The Coming White Underclass." *Wall Street Journal*, October 29.

Nathanson, Bernard. 1983. *The Abortion Papers: Inside the Abortion Mentality*. New York: Frederick Fell.

National Advisory Board on Ethics in Reproduction. 1994. "Report on Human Cloning through Embryo Splitting." *Kennedy Institute of Ethics Journal* 4: 251–82.

Nelkin, Dorothy. 1992. "The Social Power of Genetic Information." In *The Code of Codes: Scientific and Social Issues in the Human Genome Project*. Cambridge: Harvard University Press.

Nelkin, Dorothy, and M. Susan Lindee. 1995. *The DNA Mystique: The Gene as a Cultural Icon*. New York: W. H. Freeman.

Nilsson, Lennart. 1990. "The First Pictures Ever of How Life Begins" (photo essay). *Life*, August.

O'Brien, Mary. 1981. *The Politics of Reproduction*. London: Routledge.

Office of Technology Assessment. 1988. *Biology, Medicine, and the Bill of Rights*. Washington, D.C.: U.S. Government Printing Office.

Omi, Michael, and Howard Winant. 1994. *Racial Formation in the United States: From the 1960s to the 1990s*. New York: Routledge.

Overall, Christine. 1987. *Ethics and Human Reproduction: A Feminist Analysis*. Boston: Allen & Unwin.

Pateman, Carole. 1988. *The Sexual Contract*. Stanford, Calif.: Stanford University Press.

———. 1989. *The Disorder of Women: Democracy, Feminism, and Political Theory*. Stanford, Calif.: Stanford University Press.

Paul, Diane B. 1994. "Eugenic Anxieties, Social Realities, and Political Choices." In *Are Genes Us? The Social Consequences of the New Genetics*, ed. Carl F. Cranor. New Brunswick, N.J.: Rutgers University Press.

Petchesky, Rosalind. 1981. "Antiabortion, Antifeminism, and the Rise of the New Right." *Feminist Studies* 2: 206–46.

———. 1984. *Abortion and Woman's Choice: The State, Sexuality, and Reproductive Freedom*. New York: Longman.

———. 1987. "Fetal Images: The Power of Visual Culture in the Politics of Reproduction." In *Reproductive Technologies: Gender, Motherhood, and Medicine*, ed. Michelle Stanworth. Minneapolis: University of Minnesota Press.

———. 1995. "The Body as Property: A Feminist Re-vision." In *Conceiving the New World Order: The Global Politics of Reproduction*, ed. Faye D. Ginsberg and Rayna Rapp. Berkeley: University of California Press.

Phalen, Peggy. 1993. *Unmarked: The Politics of Performance*. New York: Routledge.

Phelan, Shane. 1990. "Foucault and Feminism." *American Journal of Political Science* 34: 421–40.

Phillips, Anne. 1991. *Engendering Democracy*. Cambridge: Polity.

Plato. 1977. *Timaeus*, trans. Desmond Lee. New York: Penguin.

Pollitt, Katha. 1995. *Reasonable Creatures: Essays on Women and Feminism*. New York: Vintage.

Poovey, Mary. 1988. *Uneven Developments: The Ideological Work of Gender in Mid-Victorian England*. Chicago: University of Chicago Press.

Purdy, Laura, ed. 1989. "Ethics and Reproduction" (special issue). *Hypatia* 4 (3).

Rabinow, Paul. 1992. "Artificiality and Enlightenment: From Sociobiology to Biosociality." In *Incorporations*, ed. Jonathan Crary and Sanford Kwinter. New York: Zone.

———. 1996. *Essays in the Anthropology of Reason*. Princeton, N.J.: Princeton University Press.

Rapp, Rayna. 1990. "Constructing Amniocentesis: Maternal and Medical Discourses." In *Uncertain Terms: Negotiating Gender in American Culture*, ed. Faye D. Ginsberg and Anna Lowenhaupt Tsing. Boston: Beacon.

———. 1993. "Reproduction and Gender Hierarchy: Amniocentesis in America." In *Sex and Gender Hierarchies*, ed. Barbara D. Miller. Cambridge: Cambridge University Press.

———. forthcoming. "Real Time Is Prime Time: The Role of the Sonogram in the Age of Mechanical Reproduction." In *Cyborgs and Citadels: Anthropological Interventions into Techno-Medicine*, ed. G. Downey, J. Dunit, and Sharon Traweek. Seattle: University of Washington Press.

Rayner, Alice. 1994. "Cyborgs and Replicants: On the Boundaries." *discourses* 16 (3): 124–43.

Rendall, Jane. 1987. "Virtue and Commerce: Women in the Making of Adam Smith's Political Economy." In *Women in Western Political Philosophy*, ed. Ellen Kennedy and Susan Mendus. New York: St. Martin's.

Rhode, Deborah L. 1989. *Justice and Gender: Sex Discrimination and the Law*. Cambridge: Harvard University Press.

Ritvo, Harriet. 1992. "Race, Breed, and Myths of Origins: Chillingham Cattle as Ancient Britons." *Representations* 39: 1–22.

Robertson, John A. 1986. "Embryos, Families, and Procreative Liberty: The Legal Structure of the New Reproduction." *Southern California Law Review* 59: 939–1041.

Robinson, Cherylon. 1993. "Surrogate Motherhood: Implications for the Mother-Fetus Relationship." In *The Politics of Pregnancy: Policy Dilemmas in the Maternal-Fetus Relationship*, ed. Janna C. Merrick and Robert H. Blank. Binghamton, N.Y.: Haworth.

Rorvik, David M. 1971. "Taking Life into Our Own Hands: The Test-Tube Baby Is Coming." *Look*, May 18, 83–88.

Rosenfeld, Albert. 1969. "Science, Sex, and Tomorrow's Morality." *Life*, June 13, 37–51.

Rothman, Barbara Katz. 1986. *The Tentative Pregnancy: Prenatal Diagnosis and the Future of Motherhood*. New York: Penguin.

————. 1989. *Recreating Motherhood: Ideology and Technology in a Patriarchal Society*. New York: W. W. Norton.

Rousseau, Jean-Jacques. 1979. *Emile; or, On Education*, trans. Allan Bloom. New York: Basic Books.

Rubin, Eva R. 1987. *Abortion, Politics, and the Courts: Roe v. Wade and Its Aftermath*. Westport, Conn.: Greenwood.

Russett, Cynthia Eagle. 1989. *Sexual Science: The Victorian Construction of Womanhood*. Cambridge: Harvard University Press.

Ryan, Maura A., 1990. "The Argument for Unlimited Procreative Liberty: A Feminist Critique." *Hastings Center Report* 20 (4): 6–12.

Ryan, Michael, and Avery Gordon, eds. 1994. *Body Politics: Disease, Desire, and the Family*. Boulder, Colo.: Westview.

Sacks, Oliver. 1993. "To See and Not See." *New Yorker*, May 10.

Saltenberger, Ann. 1983. *Every Woman Has a Right to Know the Dangers of Legal Abortion*. Glassboro, N.J.: Air-Plus Enterprises.

Sandelowski, Margarete. 1994. "Separate, but Less Equal: Fetal Ultrasonography and the Transformation of Expectant Mother/Fatherhood." *Gender and Society* 8: 230–45.

Sapiro, Virginia, ed. 1985. *Women, Biology, and Public Policy*. Beverly Hills: Sage.

Sarat, Austin, and Thomas R. Kearns. 1991. *The Fate of Law*. Ann Arbor: University of Michigan Press.

————, eds. 1993. *Law in Everyday Life*. Ann Arbor: University of Michigan.

Sawicki, Jana. 1991. *Disciplining Foucault: Feminism, Power, and the Body*. New York: Routledge.

"Scapegoating the Black Family." 1989. *The Nation* (special issue), July 24–31.

Scheppele, Kim Lane. 1990. "Facing Facts in Legal Interpretation." *Representations* 30: 42–77.

Schiebinger, Londa. 1989. *The Mind Has No Sex? Women in the Origins of Modern Science*. Cambridge: Harvard University Press.

————. 1993. *Nature's Body: Gender in the Making of Modern Science*. Boston: Beacon.

Schlafly, Phyllis. 1977. *The Power of the Positive Woman*. New York: Jove.

Schlutz, Marjorie M. 1991. "Reproductive Technology and Infant-Based Parenthood: An Opportunity for Gender Neutrality." *Wisconsin Law Review* 1991: 297–398.

Schneider, David M. 1980. *American Kinship: A Cultural Account*. Chicago: University of Chicago Press.

————. 1984. *A Critique of the Study of Kinship*. Ann Arbor: University of Michigan Press.

Schroedel, Jean Reith, and Paul Peretz. 1994. "A Gender Analysis of Policy Formation: The Case of Fetal Abuse." *Journal of Health Politics, Policy and Law* 19: 336–60.

Shanley, Mary Lyndon. 1993. "'Surrogate Mothering' and Women's Freedom: A Critique of Contracts for Human Reproduction." *Signs* 18: 618–38.

Sheehan, James J., and Morton Sosna, eds. 1991. *The Boundaries of Humanity: Humans, Animals, Machines*. Berkeley: University of California Press.

Shevory, Thomas. 1993. "The War at Home: Positivism, Law, and the Prosecution of Pregnant Women." In *The Politics of Pregnancy: Policy Dilemmas in the Maternal-Fetal Relationship*, ed. Janna C. Merrick and Robert H. Blank. Binghamton, N.Y.: Haworth.

Siegel, Reva. 1992. "Reasoning from the Body: A Historical Perspective on Abortion Regulation and Questions of Equal Protection." *Stanford Law Review* 44: 261–381.

Singer, Linda. 1992. *Erotic Welfare: Sexual Theory and Politics in the Age of Epidemic*, ed. Judith Butler and Maureen MacGrogen. New York: Routledge.

Singer, Peter, and William Walters, eds. 1982. *Test-Tube Babies*. Melbourne: Oxford University Press.

Singer, Peter, and Deane Wells. 1985. *Making Babies: The New Science and Ethics of Conception*. New York: Charles Scribner's Sons.

Smart, Carol. 1989. *Feminism and the Power of Law*. London: Routledge.

Snitow, Ann. 1986. "The Paradox of Birth Technology: Exploring the Good, the Bad, and the Scary." *Ms.*, December.

Solinger, Ricki. 1992. *Wake Up Little Susie: Single Pregnancy and Race before Roe v. Wade*. New York: Routledge.

Spallone, Patricia, and Deborah Lynn Steinberg, eds. 1987. *Made to Order: The Myth of Reproductive and Genetic Progress*. New York: Pergamon.

Spellman, Elizabeth V. 1988. *Inessential Women: Problems of Exclusion in Feminist Thought*. Boston: Beacon.

Stabile, Carole A. 1992. "Shooting the Mother: Fetal Photography and the Politics of Disappearance." *camera obscura* 28: 178–205.

Stange, Margit. 1994. "The Broken Self: Fetal Alcohol Syndrome and Native American Selfhood." In *Body Politics: Disease, Desire, and the Family*, ed. Michael Ryan and Avery Gordon. Boulder, Colo.: Westview.

Stanworth, Michelle, ed. 1987. *Reproductive Technologies: Gender, Motherhood, and Medicine*. Minneapolis: University of Minnesota Press.

———. 1990. "Birth Pangs: Conceptive Technologies and the Threat to Motherhood." In *Conflicts in Feminism*, ed. Marianne Hirsch and Evelyn Fox Keller. New York: Routledge.

Stark, Barbara. 1988. "Constitutional Analysis of the Baby M Decision." *Harvard Women's Law Journal* 11: 19–52.

Steinberg, Deborah Lynn. 1991. "Adversarial Politics: The Legal Construction of Abortion." In *Off-Centre: Feminism and Cultural Studies*, ed. Sarah Franklin, Celia Lury, and Jackie Stacey. New York: HarperCollins.

Stotland, Nada L. 1992. "Commentary: The Myth of the Abortion Trauma Syndrome." *Journal of the American Medical Association* 269: 2078–79.

Strathern, Marilyn. 1992. *After Nature: English Kinship in the Late Twentieth Century*. Cambridge: Cambridge University Press.

———. 1992. *Reproducing the Future: Essays on Anthropology, Kinship and the New Reproductive Technologies*. New York: Routledge.

Stumpf, Andrea E. 1986. "Redefining Mother: A Legal Matrix for New Reproductive Technologies." *Yale Law Journal* 96: 187–208.

Suleiman, Susan Rubin, ed. 1986. *The Female Body in Western Culture*. Cambridge: Harvard University Press.

Sullivan, William M. 1986. *Reconstructing Public Philosophy*. Berkeley: University of California Press.

Sumner, William Graham. 1986. *What Social Classes Owe to Each Other* (1883). Caldwel, Idaho: Caxton.

Superior Court of New Jersey, Bergen County. 1987. "In the Matter of Baby 'M.'" *Opinion*, March 31, 1–121.

Taylor, Janelle S. 1992. "The Public Fetus and the Family Car: From Abortion Politics to a Volvo Advertisement." *Public Culture* 4 (2): 67–80.

Taylor, Lucien, ed. 1994. *Visualizing Theory: Selected Essays from V.A.R. 1990–1994*. New York: Routledge.

Terry, Jennifer. 1989. "The Body Invaded: Medical Surveillance of Women as Repro-
ducers." *Socialist Review* 19 (3): 13–43.

Treichler, Paula A. 1990. "Feminism, Medicine, and the Meaning of Childbirth." In
Body/Politics: Women and the Discourses of Science, ed. Mary Jacobus, Evelyn Fox
Keller, and Sally Shuttleworth. New York: Routledge.

Tribe, Lawrence H. 1973. "Technology Assessment and the Fourth Discontinuity:
The Limits of Instrumental Rationality." *Southern California Law Review* 46:
617–60.

Tsing, Anna Lowenhaupt. 1990. "Monster Stories: Women Charged with Perinatal En-
dangerment." In *Uncertain Terms: Negotiating Gender in American Culture*, ed.
Faye D. Ginsberg and Anna Lowenhaupt Tsing. Boston: Beacon.

"The 21st Century Family." 1990. *Newsweek* (special edition), Winter/Spring.

Turner, Bryan S. 1984. *The Body and Society*. New York: Basil Blackwell.

Van Dyck, Jose. 1995. *Manufacturing Babies and Public Consent: Debating the New
Reproductive Technologies*. New York: Macmillan.

Vernant, Jean-Pierre. 1983. *Myth and Thought among the Greeks*. London: Routledge.

Vidal-Naquet, Pierre. 1988. "Aeschylus, the Past, and the Present." In *Myth and
Tragedy in Ancient Greece*, ed. Jean-Pierre Vernant and Pierre Vidal-Naquet. New
York: Zone.

Wallis, Claudia. 1984. "Making Babies: The New Science of Conception." *Time*, September 10, 46–53.

Watson-Verran, Helen, and David Turnbull. 1995. "Science and Other Indigenous
Knowledge Systems." In *Handbook of Science and Technology Studies*, ed. Sheila
Jasanoff, Gerald E. Markle, James C. Petersen, and Trevor Pinch. Thousand Oaks,
Calif.: Sage.

Whitbeck, Caroline. 1988. "Fetal Imaging and Fetal Monitoring: Finding the Ethical
Issues." In *Embryos, Ethics, and Women's Rights*, ed. Elaine Hoffman Barauch,
Amadeo F. D'Adamo Jr., and Joni Seagar. New York: Harrington Park.

White, James Boyd. 1984. *When Words Lose Their Meaning: Constitutions and Reconstitutions of Language, Character, and Community*. Chicago: University of
Chicago Press.

———. 1990. *Justice as Translation: An Essay in Cultural and Legal Criticism*.
Chicago: University of Chicago Press.

Whiteford, Linda M., and Marilyn L Poland, eds. 1989. *New Approaches to Human
Reproduction: Social and Ethical Dimensions*. Boulder, Colo.: Westview.

Whitehead, Mary Beth, with Loretta Schwartz-Nobel. 1989. *A Mother's Story*. New
York: St. Martin's.

Wiegman, Robyn. 1995. *American Anatomies: Theorizing Race and Gender*. Durham,
N.C.: Duke University Press.

Wikler, Daniel. 1984. "Abortion, Privacy, and Personhood: From Roe v. Wade to the
Human Life Statute." In *Abortion: Moral and Legal Perspectives*, ed. Jay L. Garfield
and Patricia Hennesey. Amherst: University of Massachusetts Press.

Williams, Patricia J. 1991. *The Alchemy of Race and Rights*. Cambridge: Harvard University Press.

———. 1994. "Hate Radio: Why We Need to Tune In to Limbaugh and Stern." *Ms.*,
March/April.

Willis, Ellen. 1992. *No More Nice Girls: Countercultural Essays*. Middletown, Conn.:
Wesleyan University Press.

Winner, Langdon. 1986. *The Whale and the Reactor*. Chicago: University of Chicago
Press.

Wintgerter, Rex B. 1987. "Fetal Protection Becomes Assault on Motherhood." *In These Times*, June 10–23.

Wollstonecraft, Mary. 1975. *A Vindication of the Rights of Women*, ed. Carol H. Poston. New York: W. W. Norton.

Wood, Carl, and Ann Westmore. 1983. *Test-Tube Conception*. Englewood Cliffs, N.J.: Prentice Hall.

Woodmansee, Martha, and Peter Jaszi, eds. 1994. *The Construction of Authorship: Textual Appropriation in Law and Literature*. Durham, N.C.: Duke University Press.

Yanagisako, Sylvia, and Carol Delaney, eds. 1995. *Naturalizing Power: Essays in Feminist Cultural Analysis*. New York: Routledge.

Zeitlin, Froma. 1978. "The Dynamics of Misogyny: Myth and Mythmaking in the Oresteia." *Arethusa* 11: 149–77.

Index

Petchesky, Rosalind, 36, 90
postabortion stress syndrome, 42–43, 58,
  61; appearance of, 58; evidence for,
  58–59
postmenopausal therapy and popular discourse, 89, 90, 91, 132
postmortem ventilation therapy, 26–27,
  124; and the meaning of motherhood,
  47–50
prochoice politics, 52, 53–54, 58, 59–60,
  65–66

racial difference: historical production of,
  21–22; and the reproduction of white
  prerogative, 8, 19, 94–95, 131
Ramsey, Paul, 113
Reagan, Ronald, 17, 35, 40, 86
Reagan-Bush era, 17, 86, 87, 101
Rees, Michael, 105
reproduction, narratives of, 77–79, 91–93
reproductive autonomy, 6, 49–50, 65–66,
  151 n19
reproductive freedom, 66–67, 104–5,
  131–32
reproductive technologies: contests over
  signification of, 9, 115–16, 131–32;
  and cultural transformation, 18,
  112–15; disciplining of female bodies
  through, 78, 80–82; political possibilities of, 8, 18, 49–50, 83, 97–98, 116;
  and the reinscription of dominant
  power relations, 4, 20–21, 115–16,
  130–31; as technologies of gender, 25,
  66–67, 72–73
reproductive technology: law as a, 8,
  18–21, 71–73, 86–87, 94–98, 115,
  119; science as a, 21–25, 90, 115,
  126–30
Rifkin, Jeremy, 121
Roe v. Wade, 2, 5, 33, 65
Rosenberg, Leon, 33–34

Sacks, Oliver 3, 11–13
S'Aline's Solution, 51, 58, 59, 60, 66, 67
San Francisco Chronicle, 26, 27
Sawicki, Jana, 83
seeing: and the assumed transparency of
  reality, 14, 15, 24, 39, 64; cultural logic
  and operation of, 3–4, 18–25; cultural
  work performed through, 21–25,
  61–64; and positivism, 16; situated

character of, 11–14, 17; as a social
  practice, 12–14, 63–64
semen, 21, 62, 124, 154 n31; ancient
  Greek conceptions of, 77, 146 n33
Senate Judiciary Subcommittee Hearings,
  U.S., 4–5; and Human Life Statute,
  32–34, 139 n18; and National Acad-
  emy of Science, 34
sexual difference, 21–22
sexual regulation, 2–3, 106–9, 131–32
sexuality, black female: and class, 86; and
  maternity, 45, 95–97, 106–9, 131
sexuality, white female: and class, 106–9;
  and maternity, 44, 68–69, 131
Siegel, Riva, 133–34 n10
Silent Scream, 35–37, 52, 60, 61, 90
Solinger, Ricki, 107
Steiner, William, 94
Steptoe, Patrick, 25, 44, 48, 113
Stern, Bill, 8
Stillman, Robert, 9, 116–17
Strathern, Marilyn, 132
Supreme Court, U.S., abortion decisions
  of, 1–3, 5, 33, 64–65
surrogacy, 7–8; as baby selling, 69, 70,
  86, 88; and the disruption of kinship
  structures, 19–20, 48, 71–72; gestational, 85–98; as a legal practice,
  19–20; and maternal instinct, 72, 88;
  and procreative desire, 19, 74–75; and
  the reinvention of paternal law, 78;
  traditional forms of, 73, 134 n15, 145
  n18
surrogate mother: as cultural monstrosity,
  7–8, 131–32; legal representations of,
  134–35 n16; legal status of, 8, 78–79
surveillance of maternal body, 36, 38

Three Men and a Baby, 61
Time magazine, 44, 110, 112, 113, 116,
  121

ultrasound, 23; and maternal bonding,
  36–37, 51, 89–91

Vernant, Jean-Pierre, 76
Videl-Naquet, Pierre, 76
visualizing practices: and biological
  reproduction, 38–41, 90; cultural assumptions reinforced by, 58–61, 65–66;
  and cultural reproduction, 14–17, 35;